MARATHON AND HALF MARATHON

THE BEGINNER'S GUIDE

MARATHON
AND
HALF MARATHON

MARNIE CARON
& THE SPORT MEDICINE COUNCIL OF BRITISH COLUMBIA
FOREWORD BY JACK TAUNTON, M.D.

GREYSTONE BOOKS
Douglas &McIntyre Publishing Group
Vancouver/Toronto/Berkeley

Greystone Books
A division of Douglas & McIntyre Ltd.
2323 Quebec Street, Suite 201
Vancouver, British Columbia
Canada V5T 4S7
www.greystonebooks.com

Library and Archives Canada Cataloguing in Publication

Caron, Marnie
Marathon and half marathon : the beginner's guide / Marnie Caron and the Sport Medicine Council of British Columbia ; foreword by Jack Taunton.
Includes index.
ISBN-13: 978-1-55365-158-1
ISBN-10: 1-55365-158-8
1. Marathon running–Training. I. Sport Medicine Council of B.C. II. Title.
GV1065.17.T73C37 2006   796.42'52   C2005-906669-5

Library of Congress information is available upon request

Editing by Jill Lambert
Cover design by Jessica Sullivan
Text design by Warren Clark
Cover photograph by Yellow Dog Productions/Getty Images
Printed and bound in Canada by Friesens
Printed on acid-free paper that is forest friendly
(100% post-consumer recycled paper) and has been processed chlorine free.
Distributed in the U.S. by Publishers Group West

We gratefully acknowledge the financial support of the Canada Council for the Arts, the British Columbia Arts Council, and the Government of Canada through the Book Publishing Industry Development Program (BPIDP) for our publishing activities.

Dedication

To my running companions,
and to Brad: thank you for
your generosity of spirit and
for sharing in the belief that
all things are possible.

Contents

Acknowledgments

I would like to acknowledge and give thanks to the many friends and members of the running community and sport medicine practitioners who provided direction, support, and inspiration, with special thanks to: Dr. Bryan Barootes, Lynda Cannell, Dr. Liz Joy, Lynn Kanuka, Rita King, Jill Lambert, Thom Lutes, Phil Moore, Dallas Parsons, Dr. Nicky Peterson, Dr. Trent Smith, Dr. Jack Taunton, and Dr. Whitney Sedgwick.

Foreword

RUNNING A HALF OR FULL MARATHON IS WITHIN MOST people's reach, as long as they train correctly. Going the distance takes commitment and patience, and it requires a good training program accompanied by sound advice. *Marathon and Half Marathon: The Beginner's Guide* will pilot a sedentary person from inactivity through to finishing a half marathon or full marathon in 26 weeks. It will also help those who have had a bit more experience and are looking for new challenges beyond the 10-kilometer distance.

The Sport Medicine Council of British Columbia clearly understands the unique needs of the beginning runner. Using the principles developed by physicians at the Allan McGavin Sport Medicine Centre at the University of British Columbia, SportMedBC created programs and clinics to teach new runners and walkers how to train safely and effectively for a 10-kilometer event. Ten years and three editions later, *The Beginning Runner's Handbook* is still on best-seller lists, and tens of thousands of people have benefited from training clinics or have used the programs to train on their own. I am pleased that in response to many requests, SportMedBC's Beginner's Guide series has evolved to include training for half and full marathons.

The success of the Beginner's Guide series is founded primarily on its training programs. A panel of distance-running experts, including Olympians, coaches, and running-clinic leaders, has developed sound training and coaching advice. Combined with injury-prevention tips from sport medicine specialists and nutrition advice from sport dietitians, the step-by-step plan laid out in this book is a road map for successfully completing your first half or full marathon.

As a sport medicine physician, I highly recommend SportMedBC's approach to training. The walk/run method is a safe and easy way for your body to adjust to the demands of running or jogging longer distances. Armed with this book, all you need to add is a desire to go the distance, willingness to follow the advice and tips, and a commitment to consistently stay with the prescribed training.

Along the way, of course, the multiple benefits that will accrue from following the book's principles are their own reward, whether or not you ever decide to run in an organized marathon event. But once you're achieving your goals on a daily or weekly basis, you'll probably find running a half or full marathon irresistible. Good luck with your training, and stick with it.

Jack Taunton, MD
Allan McGavin Sport Medicine Centre
University of British Columbia
Vancouver

The Mystique of the Marathon

YOU'RE DRIVING TO WORK, AND YOU WATCH FROM THE comfort of your car as the early morning light faintly illuminates three sinewy subjects. Little else is clear. One locks a bike to a tree, and two others emerge from their cars, each moving from different points toward a fountain, a meeting place for the ritual morning run. As the three women approach, their smiling faces shed light on much, much more about their characters.

Some people feel best moving in a car or a train, others while riding a bike, and a special few find their joy in running. They are a rare breed, the runners who, with the grace of gazelles, win races, medals, and accolades. These whippet-like creatures are perfectly relaxed, while perfectly active.

We're not all gazelles, and many of us won't win races. Running—especially distance running—for most of us is not something that is seamless. It is a mountain of hard work that takes patience, love, and, most of all, perseverance.

You've never done a lot of running, or walking, for that matter, or perhaps it's been a long time since you did. Either way, you're finding yourself noticing runners out on the roads at all times of the day and night. You have a nagging question for yourself: "Am I crazy, or could I actually consider trying to be one of these people? Do I dare ask how or even consider the possibility of training for a half or a full marathon?"

At one time, completing a marathon was considered to be an almost Herculean endeavor. Today, many of us know someone who has completed a marathon, but training to run a half or full marathon continues to be an extraordinary achievement. Whether it is your sister-in-law who ran 26.2 miles (42.1 kilometers) in 3:30 hours to qualify for the prestigious Boston Marathon or your colleague who crossed the finish line in 5 hours with excitement lighting his face, it is an amazing accomplishment.

With an effective program, training for and completing a distance event like the marathon in a safe and healthy manner could be a reality for you. The journey is not o-nly a great way to improve your health and fitness but also will be an experience you will never regret.

Common Questions

What is the length of each event?

The marathon is 26.2 miles, or 42.1 kilometers. The half marathon is half that distance at 13.1 miles, or 21.05 kilometers.

Why choose distance running?

Ask runners why they run and the most common reason cited is the simplicity of the activity. You can do it almost anywhere and at any time. It's also one of the least expensive sports around. Once you find a good pair of running shoes, you're basically done. Unlike running, the cost of golf, skiing, or tennis is a continuum of green fees, lift tickets, and court rentals. Also, distance running is a sport that can teach you a lot about yourself, show you your limitations, and give you the opportunity to overcome them. Distance running requires commitment, determination, desire, hard work, and a sense of self-worth. Consider how many other areas in your life would benefit from your having these attributes.

What exactly is a marathon?

A marathon is a running race over a distance officially set at 26.2 miles. It has an interesting history that dates back to 490 BC. According to Greek legend, a soldier ran to Athens from a battlefield near Marathon, Greece, to deliver the news of a Greek victory over the Persians. According to history books, he then collapsed and died of exhaustion. The story is fictionalized to some degree, but it inspired one of the world's greatest and most prestigious sporting events: the marathon. The race remained obscure until the running boom of the late 1970s to early '80s, when "fun runs" became increasingly popular.

Why the half marathon?

The half marathon is quickly becoming a popular event

Running for pleasure

The health benefits of running are far reaching. Aerobic exercise improves your:

- Heart rate
- Cardiovascular system
- Muscle tone
- Weight control
- Circulation
- Sleep patterns

for distance runners around the world. Once thought of as merely a stepping-stone en route to the marathon, it is now a significant event in and of itself. According to a 2002 issue of *Runner's World* magazine, race organizers across North America are seeing an increasing switch to the half marathon by runners who have previously completed marathons. Now, for various reasons, they don't want to commit the time and effort required for the marathon, but they still want to challenge themselves to a distance event. The growing popularity of the half marathon can also be attributed to the huge increase in the numbers of walk/runners, people who intersperse running with walking. As well, a large number of walkers, commonly also referred to as striders, are participating in half marathons.

What about walking?

Walkers are just like runners in their quest to improve health and fitness by setting their minds on the goal of completing a half marathon. Walkers are not excluded from participating in marathons, although time demands for completing the event can be off-putting. Walkers usually take at least 7 hours to complete 26.2 miles. Most marathon courses are only open for approximately 7 hours. Consequently, walkers do not receive adequate support in the final hours of the event, when they need it the most. Without aid stations, volunteers directing and managing traffic, road closures, and little or no finish-line celebration, walking a marathon route can be dangerous and less enjoyable. Not to mention that even the fittest individual would find 7-plus hours of continuous exercise incredibly demanding. In contrast, the half marathon is more approachable, taking about 4 hours or less to complete.

So who can do a half or full marathon?

Most people with proper training can successfully walk/run 13.1 or 26.2 miles. But first you might want to consider what your goals are and what they are likely to become in the future. Very few people in their first couple of years of running run a marathon without encountering some sort of injury. Second, before you start a training program for a half or full marathon, remember that it's your health and your body we're talking about. You want to be sure that you are physically and mentally up for the challenge. The following few chapters provide you with information that will help you in establishing your distance-running goals.

I'm still interested. What else do I need to think about?

1. Can I make the commitment?

It takes a huge amount of time to prepare properly. In this book we suggest 26 weeks to prepare for either the full or half marathon, with three workout sessions per week, one of which may eventually require several hours to complete.

2. Will I have support?

This kind of commitment is without doubt a lifestyle change, and those people important in your life will be part of it and affected by it.

3. Do I have limiting health concerns?

If you have, or have had, any injuries or illnesses that may interfere with your program, you need to be realistic and honest with yourself now to avoid disap-

Marty

Marty is a 45-year-old, single career woman who loves every kind of sport. An athletic girl from an early age, her first passion was softball. She was perfect for the sport, strong and agile, with great hand-eye coordination. Marty played varsity softball for a division 1 school in California and later played for the United States' National team. But after dislocating her shoulder and suffering ongoing wrist problems from years as a catcher, she decided to end her softball career. Initially, Marty kept busy with work and friends, but over the years she found herself increasingly withdrawn, choosing to spend most of her free time alone. She started to wonder if she was in more than just a funk. After sharing her concerns with a close friend, she realized that a key difference in her life was an almost complete lack of fitness. Besides the occasional walk, she was pretty sedentary, and since her softball days she hadn't experienced that post-exercise high that she loved so much. Fitness had always been a huge part of her life, so it's not surprising that she didn't feel like herself without it.

Marty's friend encouraged her to take up running. Marty agreed, and she was hooked almost instantly. Before long she found herself signing up for a half-marathon training clinic. She definitely wanted to do a full marathon one day, but given that she was new to running, she felt a slow and gradual approach was best. The clinic was close to Marty's home and she really liked her assigned training group. Unfortunately, in her second month of training she caught a terrible cold that forced her to miss 2 weeks of training. When she returned, she found the pace of her training group to be too challenging. Initially, she was discouraged and questioned her desire to train and to run a half marathon. She liked running, but she wondered if she would be happier just scrapping the half-marathon goal and running on her own. Ultimately, she chose not to make a snap decision and instead opted to train with a slower group for a week, after which time she would make a decision about the marathon. After only a couple of training sessions with her new group, Marty was more committed than ever to her half-marathon goal. In her time away while ill, she had forgotten how much she loved the comradery of sharing a common goal and a passion for her newfound sport.

Marathon and Half Marathon

pointment. Check with a sport medicine physician and explain your health care concerns before establishing your distance-running goals. It may be, for example, that you need a longer buildup to a half marathon than we recommend in the 26-week program, or possibly you should first work toward a 5- or 10-kilometer (3.1- or 6.2- mile) event.

4. Am I prepared to take care of myself?

You are embarking on a very demanding exercise program, and you'll need to ensure all aspects of your life stay on a healthy track; everything from nutrition to hydration and good sleeping patterns plays a part in a sound training program.

5. Am I mentally strong enough to physically make this happen?

The psychological barriers of the distance-running journey can be the greatest obstacles to overcome. But if you are up for the challenge, and persevere through the mental challenges of a 26-week walk/run program, you will be stronger, wiser, and know yourself a little bit better than before you started the journey.

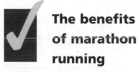

The benefits of marathon running

- Improved health
- Increased energy
- Improved self-esteem
- Time with friends
- Quality time outdoors
- Stress relief
- Weight control
- Character building

2 Getting Started

"GO BIG OR GO HOME!" "THE MARATHON IS TO RUNNERS what Everest is to climbers!" These are just a couple of the images or comparisons that come to mind when deciding between the goal of a half or full marathon. The marathon is, without question, the granddaddy of running races. It is an achievement that bestows serious bragging rights over the water cooler at work. But you have to ask yourself if this single reason—permission to boast—is enough to motivate you through 26 weeks of relentless training. This is a decision that shouldn't be taken lightly. Although blisters, chafing, and fatigue are all elements of half- and full-marathon training, the demands are significantly different.

A Safe and Effective Approach to Distance Running

From couch potato to 26.2 or 13.1 miles (42 or 21 kilometers) in 26 weeks. Sport medicine experts strongly suggest that people complete at least a 10-kilometer (6.2-mile) race and be running regularly for at least 6 to 12 months before considering a half marathon, and 12 months is the recommended time frame for a full-marathon goal. The body (muscles, bones, and ligaments) needs time to adapt to the stresses of running 26.2 miles. Many of you, however, probably have a friend, colleague, or family member who was a non-runner and who after only a few short months of training crossed the marathon or half-marathon finish line.

For many, 26 weeks seems a long time to prepare to complete a race. After all, running appears simple enough—and many approach it thinking success will come easily. Although the half- and full-marathon distances can seem daunting, beginning runners all too often become hurt or injured because they don't allow themselves an adequate amount of time to prepare, or they overtrain by working out too frequently and too intensely.

Our panel of running experts recognizes the growing interest of beginning runners in completing a marathon or half marathon in as short a period as possible. Keeping this in mind, after consulting sport medicine practitioners and distance-running experts we created a road map for beginning runners that will take you from the couch to the finish line using the safest and most direct route possible. Our experts decided that a walk/run approach is the best way for beginning marathoners to train for and complete both the half- and full-marathon events. The training schedules in this book start off slowly to help build strength, stamina, and confidence. Your focus over the next 26 weeks will be to improve your overall health and fitness while remaining injury free.

If you've ever watched a half- or full-marathon race, I'm sure you've seen people hobble across the finish line looking as if the last mile was more of a death march than a euphoric experience. It is our firm belief that finishing a distance race is one thing but finishing with some degree of grace is another. Hence, the philosophy behind this book is to live to run another day. Our goal is to have you not only make it to the finish line but also, in the weeks and months following, continue to reap the rewards of an active lifestyle.

Choosing between the Half and Full Marathon

Time—and time again. This is a key element separating the demands of the full and the half marathon. It takes almost twice as long to complete and recover from a marathon as it does from the half marathon. The following questions should help you decide your best running goal at this time:

- How long have you been maintaining a regular running routine?
- How much time do you have to commit to your exercise program?
- Does the time you have available for your next exercise endeavor match the demands that characterize the half or full marathon?
- Have you been injury free for the past few months?
- Have you enjoyed your recent running program enough to continue to increase the distance and intensity?
- Are you mentally and physically prepared to train for significantly longer periods of time?
- Do you have the commitment of family support?
- Do you realize there will be a "tired" factor that will

Why a growing number of runners view the half marathon as the perfect distance

- It is less physically demanding than the marathon.
- Recovery time is shorter.
- Time demands are more realistic.
- Risk of injury is lower.
- It's a great way to explore the challenges of distance running.
- It builds confidence before an attempt at the full marathon.
- It's mentally less taxing.
- It's a great way to increase your fitness level.

take its toll? You will probably need to be in bed earlier, and you will have less energy for other physical activities and less free time.

- Are you bored with running? Do you feel the need to try another athletic activity?

The half marathon

It is true that the marathon is a huge undertaking, but this is not to say that training for and completing a half marathon is an easy task. It isn't. It is a significant achievement in and of itself.

In recent years the half marathon has become increasingly popular. According to Running USA, in 2002 over half a million runners completed a half marathon, which is over 200,000 more participants than in 1987. The number of half marathons has also drastically increased. Many of the large marathons are now adding a half marathon to attract participants. As Allan Steinfeld, president and CEO of the New York Road Runners Association, points out, "The distance really makes sense... For some runners the half is an end point, something they peak for, and for anyone training to run a marathon, it's a perfect endurance test."

How to tell if you're ready for a marathon

Check your physical history before you decide whether a half or full marathon is for you:

- Ask yourself what your body has been through in the past. Have you, for example, been in a car accident, or been pregnant? Depending on your history, you may need to customize your stretching and strengthening program to accommodate your specific needs. For some stretching exercises, see appendix A.

- If you've been sedentary for a long period, it may take you longer to reach the start line. It's important to go at your own pace and trust your instincts. You may need to build extra weeks of training into the 26-week program outlined in this book.

- Once you start running, closely monitor the little aches and pains and seek expert advice on the best form of treatment, whether it be rest or extra strength and stretching exercises.

After considering these points, you may decide that training for a half or full marathon isn't for you, at least not right now. This might be the case if you are carrying a significant amount of extra weight, for example; you may find it is better to lose some weight and set short-term goals for yourself. Completing a 5- or 10-kilometer event in a few months' time might be more realistic, and you can keep the marathon as a more long-term goal you can build toward.

Are you physically able to walk/run long distances?

One way to decide whether you need medical supervision is to take a physical readiness test. The Canadian Society for Exercise Physiology has developed a good one, called the Physical Activity Readiness Questionnaire, or PAR-Q for short (see appendix B). If you complete the questionnaire without answering yes to any of the questions—and it's in your best interest to answer honestly—then you can probably start an exercise program without fear of hurting yourself. If, however, you answer yes to one or more of these questions, you should talk to your doctor before proceeding. If you want a more accurate assessment of your physical condition, ask your doctor to do a Physical Activity Readiness Medical Examination (PARmed-X).

Training to walk/run a distance event

Walk/running is a relatively new approach to distance training and racing that has inspired huge numbers of beginning runners to train for and complete distance events. From the beginning of time, animals and humans have combined walking and running. However, Olympic athlete, running teacher, and writer Jeff Galloway is responsible for creating some of the first training programs that incorporate the two activities. The theory is that by interspersing walk breaks throughout a run, beginners can gradually build endurance and strength to complete longer distances. Also, breaking runs into shorter segments with walk breaks makes the process appear less daunting.

Deciding Whether Age Is a Factor

It is unrealistic to make general rules and guidelines concerning the safe and acceptable distances that children and the aging population should run. Children grow and mature at different rates. Similarly, the aging process varies from one individual to the next.

How young is too young to train for a distance event?

Pediatrician Dr. Trent Smith of Kamloops, British Columbia, says there is very little scientific literature on which to base his recommendations. He also says that making age-based comments or assumptions for the teen population is fraught with difficulty. "For example, 14-year-olds vary—not all are at the same level of skeletal maturity. It is the skeletal age that primarily determines the type and likelihood of injury if one were to occur."

From a cardiovascular standpoint he is less concerned. In general, the hearts and lungs of children and youth are easily able to adapt to the stresses of jogging or running. Although they also need time to train, these systems rarely are limiting factors. However, Dr. Smith points out that young children tend to be more sprint oriented than youth and adults, and they tend to prefer short, sharp bursts of activity.

Dr. Smith suggests that though it might be okay for a sedentary adult to train to walk/run a marathon in 6 months, that is too short a time frame for *any* sedentary teen. This is especially the case if the teen is overweight, as that "further increases the risk of developing a lower-extremity overuse injury." Instead, Dr. Smith suggests a 3-month program to walk a 10-kilometer or run a 5-kilometer event. If a half or full marathon is still the goal, sedentary teens should give themselves at least a year of regular training.

The time frames suggested may seem a little conservative, but it's important to remember that safety depends on the skeletal maturity of the teen and on

 Pediatrician Dr. Trent Smith's tips about teens who want to run

- Make sure your teen has shoes that fit properly, provide good support, and have proper cushioning.
- Have a physician or a sport medicine doctor evaluate overweight kids for orthopedic problems.
- Let the child/teen decide on the sport or running event he or she wants to try. Encourage and support, don't force.
- Incorporate a mix of training surfaces. Trail running and turf running should be encouraged.
- Cross training can be invaluable, particularly for kids, as it keeps exercise fun and new.

whether there are any underlying orthopedic abnormalities (weight related or not). Dr. Smith suggests that for overweight teens, getting them active every day is a great start toward improved health and fitness. Once this happens, let teens set their next fitness goals; whether it's a half marathon or learning how to snowboard, the aim should be to have fun and enjoy the many benefits of an active lifestyle.

As for the extremely active teens who express interest in training for a half or full marathon, the fear for this group is burnout. If that happens, the American Academy of Pediatrics suggests the future adoption of a healthy, active lifestyle will be compromised. The same argument is made in many other sports. There is a risk of future disregard for the benefits of sport in some children who are pushed to be highly competitive at an early age.

How old is too old to begin distance running?

The 60-year-old master runner may be in better shape than the 18-year-old couch potato. But when it comes to physical changes, time does affect the human body. Beyond 30 years of age, adults start to lose muscle mass; after age 40, bone mass decreases. As well, tendons and ligaments, which connect muscle to bone and hold joints together, decrease in elasticity and therefore tear more easily. These are just some of the changes that affect the aging population's ability to enjoy sports. However, if you're over 40 and think you're too old to consider training for a distance event, please think again.

As most of us know by now, the health benefits associated with running are far reaching. Not only is running great for our physical health, it also does wonders for our mental health. In other words: running keeps us young both physically and mentally.

Dr. Bryan Barootes, a sport medicine physician based in Louisiana, says the benefits of distance running or any regular exercise program for beginners over the age of 50 is immense. There is a reduction of health risk factors such as cardiovascular disease, stroke, hypertension, diabetes, cancer (breast and colon), and mental illness. There is improvement in respiratory function, bone strength, muscle balance/strength, energy/psychological well-being, weight reduction, and overall quality of life. As Dr. Barootes says, "It's the cheapest prescription available!"

"All of these [benefits] increase with increased activity, but there is a bell curve effect—too much may increase some risk factors. It is like the ancient Greek philosophy—'Nothing in excess'," adds Dr. Barootes.

Tips for aging runners

Dr. Barootes recommends that beginning runners over 50 years of age should watch out for the following:

- The American College of Sport Medicine recommends fitness testing for those over the age of 45, or for those who are at risk for cardiovascular disease who have not been previously active and are undertaking a moderate to intense regime.
- It's important for these participants to follow the

gradual walk/run approach outlined in this book. Some individuals may need to go more slowly.

- If you have cardiovascular disease or other problems, such as diabetes, it is important to first receive clearance from your MD.

- Running does not cause arthritis, as so many believe. But it does put those with "abnormal" joints or pre-existing problems at greater risk of accelerating their challenges. Again, it's important to discuss your fitness plans with your physician prior to commencing an intense program.

- Older individuals may be more sensitive to advances in the training plan and need to "listen" to their bodies and respond accordingly. This group is most susceptible to overuse problems, particularly if they have pre-existing biomechanical problems.

- Stretching and strength training should be included in your fitness program. Cross training activities such as non-weight-bearing activities are a great way to improve strength and reduce the risk of injury and fatigue often associated with the high-impact sport of running.

Age will continue to be a debated factor in distance running, but it's important to remember that many elite marathoners don't run their first marathon until their late 20s or even early 30s. Even if you are not an elite athlete and don't want to race, the more time you train before running this distance, the more ready your body will be to handle this type of stress. If you are over the age of 30 and have had limited exposure to running and fitness, you need to check with your health care provider to ensure training for a half or full marathon is a safe and healthy goal.

Choosing Your Marathon Equipment

Most people can get away with wearing their favorite T-shirt, some cotton shorts, and an old pair of runners for a 10-kilometer run or an evening walk around the neighborhood. But a marathon is a different story. Shoes that provide good support and cushioning, as well as quick-drying and free-moving clothing that fits well and works with the environment, are key ingredients for successful preparation for the marathon itself. A marathoner's shoes and clothing can define his or her training experience as something fraught with misery and pain or full of fun and bliss.

What you wear should be primarily a function of weather and comfort. The following few pages attempt to answer the most common running-gear questions specific to marathoners.

Running shoes

Footwear has come a long way in the past 20 years, and today's modern shoes can not only help counter various foot flaws but also absorb a lot of shock.

When you run, each foot strikes the ground somewhere between 800 and 1,200 times per mile (500 and 750 times per kilometer). According to Phil Moore, owner of LadySport in Vancouver, B.C., "In the beginning, you will be coming down on your feet with one and one-half to two times your body weight, but when

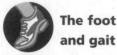

The foot and gait

Foot mechanics are broken down into three major categories:

1. The cavus-rigid (high-arched) supinator
2. The "normal" foot
3. The excessive pronator

Find a running-shoe store in your neighborhood. Good shoe retailers can suggest the various gear options to best meet your needs. They can help you find shoes that fit your profile and actually do what they are designed to do; just because a shoe is profiled for certain mechanics does not mean it will deliver those when it comes to your foot. A keen, educated, and experienced eye goes a long way to help you make a sound choice when it comes to your runners.

you get faster the impact can increase to four times your body weight. For that reason alone, your footwear needs increased cushioning throughout, particularly in the heel." It also has to provide good support for the foot and arch. Women should remember that they generally have narrower feet than men and might have trouble fitting securely into shoes designed for men. Every good running-shoe company now offers separate styles for men and women. As well, many offer shoes in various widths.

Foot numbness

Shoes that are too narrow (too tight) can cause numbness in the foot. Here are some ways to avoid this:

- Don't choose shoes that are too narrow, and don't lace them up too tightly over the instep to support the midfoot or to reduce heel slippage.
- Bear in mind that enough shoe width for a 40-minute run may cause numbness over a 3-hour period.
- Tie your shoes to give you sufficient tightness for support, especially if you are an excessive pronator, but not so snugly that you lose feeling in your toes.

Toes

Your toes will take some abuse from the long distances, and this may result in a variety of ailments. Shoes that are too short can cause black or bruised toes. A shoe that was of suitable length for a 10-kilometer run will likely be too short for a marathon or even a half marathon. Feet tend to swell over distance and time. If the foot does not have at least a thumb's width of space

Tips for selecting shoes

- When you find a shoe that works for you, don't switch just because you're curious. New isn't necessarily better—by sticking to the same brand and model, you minimize the chances of blisters, heels slipping, and other problems common to ill-fitting runners.
- If you're unsure whether it's time to buy a new pair of runners, take your shoes into your local running store and put on one old shoe and one new shoe. If the foot with the old one feels as if you have a flat tire, it's likely time to get new shoes. If it still feels okay, and there isn't a noticeable difference between your two feet, your old shoes still have some miles left.
- Marathon training will require an incredible amount of time on your feet. For beginners, the training is significantly more demanding than preparing for a 5- or 10-kilometer event. The time spent on your feet requires a shoe that can meet the demands placed on all parts of your feet, so take your time in finding a pair of shoes that work for you, and remember to replace the old ones once the cushion and support no longer feel like what you need.

between the longest toe and the end of the shoe, it is likely that the big toe and often the second toe will suffer some trauma. Shoe measurement should be taken while standing with full weight on the foot being measured.

Toenails

Trauma to the toenails comes on quickly, often without warning, and then it's too late. It results in pain, eventual loss of nails, and sometimes infection. There are occasions when the nail goes black even when there is lots of shoe length, and the nail never seems to be anywhere near the end of the shoe. This commonly happens to the four smaller toes and can be a real mystery. If the toe is clawed somewhat, it makes the nail push down into the inside of the shoe. Over short distances it may be nothing, or it may create a small blister at the end of the affected toe. Over a long distance, the nail is traumatized to the point where it creates a bleed under the nail, or "black toe." Toes that overlap can be problematic as well, creating blisters or even cuts if the nails are not kept short enough.

Nicole

Nicole, an active 30-year-old who ran a few times a week, always knew that one day she would run a marathon. For her, the marathon epitomized running. When she learned the London Marathon had selected her employer, Outward Bound, as the 2002 official charity for the race in London, England, she saw this as the perfect time to reach for her running goal while raising some much-needed funds for Outward Bound. Nicole is one of the many dedicated employees of Outward Bound, a non-profit organization that teaches life and survival skills to participants of all ages.

Over the years, the London Marathon has established itself as a premium fundraising event, selecting a different charity each year. Tens of thousands of marathoners take up the challenge to raise money for a charity that's near to their hearts. In 1998, for example, approximately 75 percent of participants in the race also raised money for the official charity.

In preparation, Nicole developed her own running program and took a relatively casual approach to preparing for the 26.2-mile event. Her relaxed attitude was the result of her busy work schedule and her manageable fundraising goal for the event. On race day, Nicole's husband and friends were along the course to cheer her to the finish. She found the first 20 miles to be pretty painless, but, like many marathoners, she struggled during the last 6 miles. Nicole felt pretty beaten up by the end, but she was able to celebrate her numerous achievements: running the entire course, finishing in her 4:30 goal time, and raising over £1,000 for Outward Bound.

At the finish of the marathon, Nicole swore she would never run another. Now that a few years have passed, she's beginning to consider another marathon, but this time she plans to follow a more detailed training program, with the goal of breaking 4 hours.

Shoes to suit your feet

- "Pronation" is the flattening of your foot's arch during weight-bearing activity such as running. The foot naturally rolls inward. It is normal to have some pronation in order for your foot to absorb shock. However, excessive pronation will put stress on your foot, as well as on other parts of your body.

- "Supination" is the opposite of pronation. It occurs when the arch does not flatten out enough during weight-bearing activity. It's less common for your foot to supinate than to pronate. If you do supinate, you will tend to walk on the outside edges of your feet.

- The "normal" foot requires a stability shoe, with moderate control features and a semi-curved inner sole.

- The "flat" foot needs a motion-control or stability shoe, with a firm midsole and a straight or semi-curved inner sole.

- The high-arched foot is best in a cushioned shoe with good flexibility. Avoid motion-control shoes with a curved inner sole.

Clothing

In the past 10 years there have been tremendous improvements in running and exercise clothing. Today, technical athletic clothing is primarily made of synthetic fibers, and you can find lightweight running shirts, sport bras, shorts, and tights made from multiple layers of nylon- and polyester-based materials. Phil Moore says, "The weaves and textures of these fabrics are designed to wick moisture away from the skin, rather than absorbing it into the garment itself. Cotton, on the other hand, can absorb up to seven times its weight in water, resulting in clothing that is colder in winter, warmer in summer, and very heavy when wet."

Consider the weather

If you're lucky enough to live in a climate that's neither too hot nor too cold, you should avoid overdressing. Your body will heat up when you run, and a jacket that's cozy when you start out will feel suffocating when you reach running temperature. When you overheat, you tend to lose a lot of body fluid through sweat, thereby dehydrating yourself. When you begin your run, you should feel a little chilly and a need to get moving.

Bill

Bill, 27, is a policy analyst for a left-wing think tank. He had been running since high school and usually managed to run three or four times per week. When he was relocated to a new city and promoted to a more demanding position within his organization, he gradually started to skip his regular runs. Between looking for a new apartment, attending dinner meetings, and being unfamiliar with the neighborhood, he seemed to have more excuses than reasons to run.

After several months of minimal exercise, Bill realized he no longer felt like himself—he had less energy, and he missed the feelings associated with running. It was at this point that he decided to join a running group: it would be a good way to meet new people, explore his new surroundings, and get motivated. The only running group available at his local community center was a half-marathon clinic. Bill had never contemplated training for a distance event, because he was certain he would not enjoy the long runs, let alone the actual race. But he was starting to feel a little desperate for some running partners and a means to motivate him to get moving. The following Sunday, he joined 20 other intermediate runners for a 70-minute trail outing at the local college.

After his first session, he was surprised at how quickly the time passed. Between the changing terrain of the trails and the constant chatter of the group, the run was more enjoyable than he had thought possible. He continued with his weekly long runs with the group, and he managed to get out for two or three lunch-hour runs during the week. In the months leading up to the half marathon, Bill began to look forward to the long run more and more. He found the pace relaxing, and he liked the feelings of satisfaction and elation at the end of each of these runs. On race day, he ran most of the distance with a couple of his new training companions. Bill was more excited than he had anticipated at completing his race goal, and he was equally happy to have met new friends and discovered his passion for long runs.

Within the first 5 to 10 minutes of warming up, you'll find you're dressed appropriately. It's a good idea to layer clothes so that you can adjust the layers to suit weather conditions.

Sport bras

Female runners will probably want to consider a sport bra, as physical activity causes the breasts to bounce. The breast is supported by a fragile structure of skin and ligaments that can be stretched by bouncing, leading to breast sag. Most everyday bras will not stop this bouncing. Enter the sport bra.

The importance of a good-fitting sport bra cannot be overstated. There are numerous types on the market,

 Tips from an elite athlete:
Stay warm in winter

Three-time Olympic rower Derek Porter uses running and skate skiing as a means to stay fit. In order to keep warm and dry during the winter months, he makes sure that his first layer of clothing is made from a technical fabric that will draw moisture away from his skin. He cautions runners to avoid cottons, as they tend to absorb moisture, leaving you damp and chilly.

Quick-drying clothing

Cotton is a great natural fabric that is good for casual clothing and bedsheets, but these days, with all the advancements in "breathable" fabrics, cotton has no place in your marathon wardrobe! If you're tempted to pull on your favorite cotton T-shirt from college before heading out the door for a long marathon-training run, just remember that cotton can absorb up to seven times its weight in water, and, when damp, can cause chafing and

lead to blisters and abrasions. As well, clammy items against your skin will make you cold in the winter.

When choosing your running gear, the most important clothing consideration is to ensure that the layer closest to your skin is nylon- or polyester-based moisture-wicking material. There are numerous great brands on the market; try a few, and pick one that fits you and your pocketbook.

Keep odors away

As a two-time Olympic triathlete, Jill Savege seems to always be changing from one sport to the next, which means she needs to use a lot of different gear. To keep her clothes smelling fresh, she washes her quick-drying fabrics regularly. "The material is great, but it is highly prone to capturing body oils and making you unpopular in close quarters. And avoid drying your running clothes next to extreme heat, like hot dryers, radiators, and campfires."

which can be confusing. Before you purchase one for your marathon training, here are a few things to consider:

- If you are large breasted, you will probably need to wear a bra that is the same size as your regular bra, rather than a "bra top," which is worn as a bra and an outer garment at the same time.

- The true supportive sport bra is usually an under-garment, which is sold by chest and cup size. Material is patterned to support in certain areas and is designed to wick away moisture.

- The elasticized lower portions of the bra, or the underwire area, need to be comfortable. Lubri-cating the area may create more problems than it solves, if the gel absorbs into the garment.

- Duct tape on the skin is a terrific anti-chafing device for all areas of the body. It is particularly good because it doesn't lose its stickiness when intro-duced to moisture.

- The shoulder straps are another common area of concern, as they can cut into the skin and/or chafe. Some bras have padded straps, or padding can be added if the bra of choice has only thin straps.

3 What's Involved?

THE BASIS OF THE TRAINING PROGRAMS IN THIS BOOK IS to build a strong foundation of walk/running. Nothing fancy; just back-to-back weeks of progressive training and a slow increase in running time that will improve your endurance and gradually develop the mental and physical strength required to complete the 13.1- or 26.2-mile (21- or 42-kilometer) course.

What most beginners may not understand is that training for a distance event like the marathon is a process of stress and rest. The programs here have you completing two short-to-medium-length sessions and one long session per week. Most sport medicine practitioners suggest that beginning marathoners should not walk/run every day and should avoid back-to-back training days. Allowing yourself one recovery day after each session increases the likelihood that you will be rested and ready for your next run, and in turn this decreases your chances of injury and overtraining.

Dealing with the Physical and Psychological Demands

Physical demands

There is no doubt that distance running is a physically demanding sport. Even the lean and fit need time to adapt to and recover from the miles of running. For the average person, or for those of you carrying some extra weight, a gradual training schedule that incorporates flexibility as well as rest and recovery days is essential.

This book does not, in any way, support the theory of "no pain, no gain." But it is important for you to understand that some level of fatigue, stiffness, and soreness is unavoidable when you begin running. As you can tell by reviewing the training program, progressing at a slow rate helps to minimize the aftereffects of running. A gradual approach also minimizes the risk of injury and burnout. The goal is to gradually and safely improve your aerobic cardiovascular fitness as well as the efficiency of your heart and lungs. The training guidelines suggested are by no means rigid. Rather, they are intended to be flexible and adaptable for the individual. We do, however, strongly encourage a graduated approach to training and discourage jumping ahead and cutting your training short of the suggested program. As we will discuss in chapter 4, if you cut your program short, you are preparing yourself for failure. You may be cheating yourself by drastically increasing the risk of injury or simply increasing the likelihood that you will fall short of your goal.

One of the biggest risks for new runners is doing too

much, too soon, and too intensely. The result is stiffness and soreness. In the early stages of your program, and possibly after some of the longer runs, you will experience some degree of muscle and joint soreness. As you get used to running, your strength and stamina will improve, and you will more easily cope with the jarring that accompanies running. As discussed, good-quality running shoes are essential to minimizing muscle and joint soreness, as is your choice of terrain. Harder surfaces such as roads, pavement, and sidewalks will likely lead to sore legs. Grass and dirt trails are softer and therefore more forgiving on the legs and muscles. As for hills: running downhill is extremely jarring on the legs. For beginning runners, it's probably best to run on flat surfaces whenever possible, and when you do have to go downhill, try to back off a bit and run extra slowly to look after your legs.

Mental and psychological demands

The mental benefits of a regular running program are immense. Some of these include confidence building, stress relief, and an overall attitude boost. And running can help train the mind as much as it can train the body. It provides an avenue to overcome the obstacles that running brings, and it is a great way to learn and to improve focus and determination. However, the mental and psychological rewards that come with distance running are hard earned. It takes time, energy, and a great deal of patience.

As chapter 6 outlines in detail, training for a marathon has significant psychological demands. In fact, many marathoners consider the mental side as demanding as the physical requirements. Distance running is an activity that requires discipline and willpower. Especially in the initial stages of your training, it can be difficult to overcome the feeling of discomfort. Discomfort—how much and how you handle it—varies from one individual to the next. Although there are countless benefits to becoming fitter and more active, it is important to understand that a marathon or half-marathon goal requires considerable mental, emotional, and psychological commitment. Turn to chapter 6 to learn more about the psychological aspect of distance running. Athletes experience highs and lows in meeting specific time or distance goals and suffering through injury or fatigue; the brain can also experience the lows of cold weather, injury, and fatigue as well as euphoria after climbing a steep hill.

Pros and Cons of Shorter Running Programs

Not every marathon or half-marathon training program is the same. Programs can vary in duration, the number of weekly training days, the recommended distance, and the suggested training pace.

At first glance, it may seem that, for example, a 13-week program would achieve the same outcome as a 26-week program but take you half the time. However, the shorter program may be just that: shorter. It takes a significant amount of time to gradually build the strength and endurance needed to complete a marathon in a safe and healthy manner. There is a stark contrast between hobbling across the finish line or never making it to the start because you're plagued by injuries, and a euphoric finish with minimal soreness and fatigue.

Sport medicine physician Dr. Jack Taunton, of the University of British Columbia's Allan McGavin Sport Medicine Centre in Vancouver, recommends that people run regularly for at least a year before training for a half or full marathon. He does recognize that an increasing number of athletes use the half or full marathon as motivation to start a regular exercise program. Understanding that this is a growing phenomenon, we have created a gradual and progressive walk/run program to get you off the couch and to the finish line in 26 weeks. The programs included in this book were designed by our panel of sport medicine practitioners, program experts, and distance-running experts to assist you in meeting your distance-running goals.

Planning Your Schedule

Exercise is like most things in life: it needs to be considered a priority in order for it to get done. If running is new to you, one of the first things you need to do is to make it part of your routine. Review your weekly schedule and decide the best times available in your week for you to run. It's important to consider the other commitments that take up your time, such as family, work, sleep, travel, and other activities. Once you have a good idea of your schedule, figure out where you can set times during the week to train. But it's important to be realistic. For example, early morning workouts are great

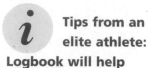
for some, but if you have difficulty functioning in the morning, a lunchtime run might be more sensible. It's not important when you do your runs, just that you set aside the time and make it a priority. By writing these times into your calendar, just as you would a work commitment, you have a much greater chance of sticking to your plans.

Keeping a Logbook

Many fitness enthusiasts and athletes have daily training records that date back 10 years or more. These records allow athletes to see the big picture and the patterns that emerge only over time. In a nutshell, your logbook will enable you to analyze the effect of your distance-running training, monitor progress, keep track of any aches and pains, help you to stay motivated, and act as a resource in the event of any injury or illness.

Consider jotting down notes about your diet in your training log. Having a record of food intake can help you identify problem times, moods, or stresses that affect your eating. And you'll be able to see how all of these things affect your training.

Robin

Robin, 35, is a product manager for a large on-line gambling company. He is also an elite runner. Originally from the East, he made the decision to leave his job with a large accounting firm and moved to the West Coast, where the climate was more conducive to training. Working part-time at a running store, Robin decided to give himself two years to focus on running to see what results he could produce. He had always been a middle-distance runner, with a personal best of 31:30 over 10 kilometers. In looking for a new challenge, he set his sights on a half marathon, 21 kilometers.

Today, years after his half-marathon debut, Robin flips through his old training logs to explain what went wrong. "In preparing for the half marathon, I see now that I didn't take the time to put the jam on top of the peanut butter. I was young, impatient, and I did too much quality and quantity (faster interval work and extremely long runs) alongside poor nutrition. I also didn't give myself enough time to increase the distance of my long run and ignored fatigue and signs of illness. On race day, I had nothing in the tank by mile 10, and instead of dropping out, I forced myself to finish the race. Two weeks after the half marathon, I became extremely sick. I wasn't the same for a couple of years afterward."

Robin was diligent in recording the details of his training: he logged the date, route, effort, type of workout, sickness, injury, and total distance, as well as weekly and monthly distance totals. Logbooks are great motivators, because at the end of the day you have to answer to your book; if you haven't run, you have to record a zero. But, as Robin points out, "They can be a double-edged sword. Logbooks police you to stay honest with your training, but it can easily become a competition between you and your book—always a challenge to see how many more miles you can record this week compared with last week. And they can also discourage cross training and rest days in order to meet your mileage goals."

It's like most things in life: if you keep your logbook in perspective, it can motivate and provide good historical value. If it weren't for Robin's logbook, he would have had a much more difficult time analyzing what went wrong in his training so that he could learn from his mistakes. He's back on track with his running, and though he doesn't have any half marathons in the foreseeable future, he is training for the upcoming cross-country season and thinks that one day he will again consider a half marathon.

Warming Up

Warming up is not just for beginners—even world-class athletes need to warm up before every workout. The purpose of a warm-up routine is to prepare your body for exercise. (Warming up itself should not be thought of as exercise, even if the routines are called warm-up "exercises.") Cold muscles work less efficiently and are more easily injured. They lack the flow of blood necessary to do the work.

Your warm-up should include some kind of general body movement designed to get the blood flowing. After about 10 minutes of moving your arms, legs, and trunk continuously, you can proceed to some gentle stretching, and the emphasis here is on *gentle*. Wendy Epp, a sport physiotherapist and competitive runner and triathlete, points out that research shows you're more likely to pull a cold muscle by stretching too vigorously than by actually starting right into jogging. "It's important to warm up progressively. A low-intensity, rhythmic activity like gentle jogging, which takes your muscles through a limited range of motion, will increase muscle and body temperature gradually and thus minimize the risk of injury."

The rule with stretching, before, during, and after exercise, is to listen to your body: if it hurts, you've gone too far. This is true regardless of how fit you are or how fast you run. You might find it annoying to get a running injury, but just imagine how frustrated you'd feel if the injury resulted from something you thought you were doing to avoid being injured! In general, runners and walkers should focus on their hamstring, calf, hip flexor, and lower-back muscles. Hold each stretch for about 10 seconds and repeat two to three times per muscle group.

Cooling Down

Just as a warm-up is the best way to prepare your body for increased levels of activity, a cooling-down procedure is the best way to ease it back down to idle speed. It's a good idea to keep your muscles active for 10 to 15 minutes after exercising, using a similar but less intense version of exactly the same thing you did during your warm-up. It takes your body and heart time to recover.

Eventually you'll find that the nice warm muscles you developed during your training session are more pliable, and that makes your post-exercise period a perfect time to work on your flexibility. After your training session, when you are thoroughly warmed up, you can safely hold each stretch for anywhere from 30 seconds to 3 minutes.

Your Training Schedule

Keep in mind that your training schedule is flexible. It's up to you to decide on which days of the week you will do each of your runs. However, it makes sense to space your runs through each week. If you're not part of a running clinic, you may also want to consider meeting a friend who runs at a similar pace for the occasional run. This helps with motivation and can make training more fun. Chapter 8 has detailed information on running clinics and training partners.

Maintenance runs/regular runs

There needs to be room in your training program for days that are for easy jogging. You will notice that the training programs outlined in this book include two runs a week that are approximately half the distance of your long run and are done at approximately the same pace as your long run. It is especially important for beginners to schedule these runs in the middle of the week to increase your comfort level when running and to allow your body to gradually adapt to the physical and mental demands of the sport.

The long run

The long run is what many marathoners and distance runners refer to as the bread and butter of their training program. "Running long" helps build cardiovascular fitness, familiarizes the body with the increased stress that comes with long-distance running, and prepares you mentally for the 26.2- or 13.1-mile course.

It seems obvious, but in order to complete a distance event like the marathon, you have to, eventually, be able to walk/run the distance. Don't be overly concerned. You will increase the distance of your long run gradually as you progress through your training program. If you turn to the section of this book that outlines your training program, you will notice that we have suggested running times as well as specific distances. Take a drive and measure the various running routes using your car's odometer. It is important to gradually build your mental and physical strength. By measuring the distance of your training runs, you avoid overtraining (running farther than necessary).

The once-a-week long run is done at a slower pace than your other sessions, so that you finish your runs feeling strong and as though you could do more. For example, if you are a 10-minute miler, you slow your long-run pace to 11 or 12 minutes per mile or even slower. The regular runner will be aware of his or her pace; if you don't know what your pace is, go to a measured track and time yourself, or measure a mile or kilometer when you are out researching your various running routes for your long run.

The pace for your first-time experience is irrelevant. It's all about respecting and preparing for the distance. Each session will bring you closer to covering the half- or full-marathon distance. On race day, you will then have the knowledge, confidence, and peace of mind that you need to complete the race.

It's important to think ahead and properly prepare yourself for your weekly long run. The shorter sessions may seem a breeze, but once you start increasing the distance of your long runs, you will soon find out that covering 16 miles is significantly more demanding mentally and physically. You can be out on your long runs for 3, 4, and sometimes 5 hours, which leaves even the fittest person fatigued. For some, the fatigue can be the result of inadequate carbohydrate stores, and for others it can be the result of dehydration. The point is that your experience is unique and might be significantly different from your training partner's. Each runner needs to assess his or her own preparation in the areas that are controllable. For example, you can certainly regulate your fluid and food intake prior to and during

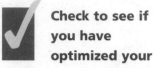

Check to see if you have optimized your long-run preparation

- Did you get enough rest the day before?
- Did you eat appropriately all week?
- Did you eat at the right times during your run?
- Did you drink enough fluids the day and evening before?
- Did you properly hydrate during the long run?
- Were you mentally prepared?
- Did you wear the best clothing for the weather conditions?
- Did you schedule your run for the best day of the week?
- Did you allow yourself enough time for the run?
- Did you organize to have a running partner join you for part or all of your run?

your sessions, and you can work to use the psychological tools you have learned.

If you're unsure whether you're going too fast on your long runs, try using distance-running guru and author Jeff Galloway's checklist. If any of the following describe you, you need to slow down:

- Following your long run, all you want to do is lie on the couch for a few hours.
- Your legs are tired and/or your muscles are sore for a few days following the long run, making it uncomfortable to run.
- You experience aches and/or pains for several days afterward.
- You are so winded during the final few miles of your long run that you cannot speak more than a few consecutive sentences.
- You feel nauseated and/or irritated at the end of the run.

A final word of caution regarding the long run: it is inevitable that for the duration of your marathon training you will have at least one extremely difficult or bad long run. This happens to everyone, even the elite. What's important is that you learn from this experience. You may be unable to pinpoint the exact cause, but the following are common factors that contribute to making a long run more painful that it needs to be:

- Dehydration
- Hunger from insufficient fueling, either before or during your run
- Walk breaks that were too short and/or too fast

- General fatigue due to the demands of work and family, or because your weekly runs were too close to your long run, giving you insufficient recovery time
- Pace that was overly aggressive

Running USA's Web site says that in 2004 the average marathon time for men was 4:23:35 and 4:55:21 for women.

Rest and recovery

Rest and recovery days are just as important in your marathon program as your training days. If you don't allow yourself enough time to recover after each run, you will not get fitter; you will just get more tired. You need to rest and recover in order to get stronger and improve. Running puts incredible demands on the body. Our half- and full-marathon programs do not have you running every day. Schedule in your rest days, just as you do your run days. Avoid running every day; spread your training sessions throughout the week. Although we have outlined a schedule for you, it is also important that you get to know your own body. Avoid being a slave to the program—be flexible, and respond to what your body is telling you.

There will be times throughout your training program when you feel run-down, fatigued, or sick with the flu or a cold, causing you to run less or occasionally miss a session. This is all part of getting to know your body. The more you run, the more you will understand what your body is telling you. It takes time to distinguish between extreme fatigue that accompanies a difficult

Tips from an elite athlete: Recover before you resume

As the bronze medal winner in the 3,000-meter track-and-field event at the 1984 Olympics in Los Angeles, Lynn Kanuka knows a little about staying healthy. Here she provides some tips for distance runners:

- If you feel stiff, tired, and sore for a day or two following a run, take more time to recover before you resume running.

- Missing a session or two doesn't mean you need to do more the following day to catch up—that is how you will get injured. Just restart your schedule when you are able to.

- Don't run every day. Remember to schedule your rest days—and stick to it!

- Spread out your training sessions throughout the week to avoid injury and overtraining.

- Patience is the key to running success. You will not improve overnight. Start cautiously and progress gradually.

session and general stiffness and soreness. Because tiredness, and sometimes soreness, usually peaks 48 hours after a run, it's good to spread out your runs. If you are still feeling sore the next time you are scheduled to run, take an extra day off. Take a walk, or try some non-weight-bearing cross training outlined in chapter 7; leave the run for the following day. The key to avoiding overuse injuries is to plan your workouts and to remain flexible in order to respond to what your body is telling you. For more on injury prevention, refer to chapter 9.

Building and reducing

Marathon and half-marathon training is draining, both mentally and physically. Regular rest days do not provide a sufficient break for your mind and body to recover over the course of a 6-month marathon-training program. In order to reduce the risk of injury, mental burnout, and reduced motivation, we have included a rest week every fourth week.

The training programs included in this book use a 4-week cycle. The first 3 weeks of every cycle gradually increase the distance of the long run, with the fourth week being a rest week. Every fourth week, the distance of your long run is reduced by approximately one-third. Even elite marathoners progress through training cycles that include a period of building followed by a shorter period of reduced volume and intensity. The rest weeks allow time to relax and provide the much-needed mental and physical break from the sometimes-grueling intensity of marathon training.

Other events

It's often a good idea to include a couple of 5- or 10-kilometer races as part of your training preparation. These races will provide you with priceless race-day experience. They will give you the opportunity to iron out some of the kinks in your pre-race-day preparations and to experience first-hand the start-line jitters, running in a crowd, taking in liquids at the aid stations, and much more. Once you've done a couple of races, you will feel more comfortable and confident in this new environment, which will reduce anxiety in the days and hours leading up to your event.

Pacing

Pacing is the process of finding a pace you can maintain throughout your training run. This is not as easy as it sounds; finding the right pace can be difficult. All too often, beginning runners take the "no pain, no gain" approach. But in the early stages of training, or when participating in events, it's important to go slowly and remember that running too fast can lead to fatigue and, possibly, physical breakdown. Give yourself the talk test. If you can speak four or five consecutive sentences without feeling winded, you are going at a pace that is good for you. If this is not the case and you feel out of breath after two sentences, you need to back off and reduce your pace.

Stay Safe

The question of safety is an issue that all female runners face. Running has many great benefits, but we cannot deny the troubling reality that women continue to be physically harmed while running. Constable Rachel Bourne of the Victoria Police Department in British Columbia suggests the following precautions to stay safe:

- Make sure you carry identification.
- Avoid dark alleys, poorly lit streets, and unpopulated areas (if you live in a city).
- Carry a cell phone in a waist pouch, or coins to make an emergency call.
- Before heading out the door on your run, be sure to tell a friend or family member where you will be running.
- Vary your route and the time of day you train. You don't want to be too predictable.
- Avoid wearing any music device, such as an iPod or MP3 player. You need to be aware of your surroundings at all times.
- Don't wear jewelry. It can attract unwanted attention.
- Trust your intuition. Avoid any person or area that feels unsafe.
- Call the police immediately if something happens to you or to someone else, or if you are being followed or harassed.

Your Running Style

As a beginning runner, technique is not something you need to worry about. Everyone, even elite runners, have idiosyncrasies or quirks that detract from their optimum pace. In time your body will gradually adopt the technique best suited to you. This is not to say that good technique doesn't pay off.

As you increase your running distance, the amount of energy lost because of poor running technique becomes more of an issue. So if you are training for a distance event, keep in mind the following tips:

- Watch that your upper body does not over-rotate or twist from side to side.
- Your arm swing should be just as comfortable as if you were walking, swinging a little away from you on the back side to just in front of your thigh in the front.
- Try to stay relaxed. If your shoulders are relaxed, the rest of your body will follow suit.
- Make sure you maintain good posture by keeping your chest cavity open; do this by not hunching forward.

If you find this difficult to envision, don't worry about your form—being relaxed is even more important. Most people should avoid tension for at least two reasons: first, tight muscles may be more susceptible to injury. Second, it takes a lot of energy to stay tense; relaxing helps channel that energy into running. While you're following your half- or full-marathon program, try to think about relaxing, assuming good posture (open your chest cavity by not hunching forward), and putting one foot in front of the other.

Where to Run

One of the great things about running is that you can do it practically anywhere—on a road, in a park, around a track, across the country, or on the spot. Nonetheless, if you have a choice, running on softer surfaces will reduce the stress and strain on bones, ligaments, tendons, and muscles and make your run more enjoyable all-round.

As a running surface, asphalt is preferable to concrete. Dirt is better yet, because it will absorb more of the impact. If concrete, which does not absorb any impact, is the worst surface, grass or rubberized tracks are probably the best, mainly because they absorb the most. Some runners find tracks boring. On the other hand, grass can hide holes or tree roots that can trip you. Consider your options carefully.

Out-and-back runs are great because:

- They teach you how to maintain an even pace.
- You learn about the dangers of going out too fast.
- It's motivating to make it to the turnaround point and know you're halfway to the end of your run.
- Knowing the route will give you increased confidence for the last, and often the most taxing, portion of your run.

If you are training for a half or full marathon that is on pavement, and you do most of your training on soft terrain, it's important to do some hard-surface running to prepare your legs for what race day will feel like.

When to Run

You've probably overheard runners remark that one of the best aspects of running is that you can do it anywhere and at any time of the day or night. Keeping safety in mind, especially for women, it's important to learn what works best for you. Of course you can do both morning and evening running, but when you plan your training schedule and organize your life accordingly, you should have a good sense of what works best for you.

Morning running

Morning runs may take you a little longer to loosen up, given that you've just got out of bed. But running at the start of your day usually increases the likelihood of sticking with a program. Too often life gets hectic, and by the end of the day our running time is competing with the demands of work and family. If you are like many people and find it difficult to function in the morning, perhaps running at noon or in the evening is a better choice.

Evening running

Many people enjoy evening runs because they feel better then than they do first thing in the morning, and they have more time. One thing to consider when running in the evening or at night is the time it will take you to cool down and wind down after your run. It's likely that you will find it difficult to sleep shortly after you finish your run.

It makes sense to schedule your long-run days when

you have the most available time: weekends, or days when you're not working, are often best.

The Programs

Initially, each training session is broken down into 5-minute components. These blocks are long enough to lead to improvement, but not so onerous that you will feel exhausted or sore. There's a psychological benefit, as well: the tasks in each block are relatively easy to complete, which will give you the confidence to graduate to the following week.

Study the programs carefully to see where you will be going and how long it will take you to get there. It's important to remember that the times noted for the training sessions do not include the time you will have to spend warming up and cooling down. For most of the program, the 5-minute blocks are divided into walking and running; as the weeks pass, the ratio of running to walking increases. For more information, turn to chapter 4. You may start to feel quite comfortable with the workouts in the early stages of your marathon program, but don't be tempted to jump ahead. Your bones, ligaments, tendons, and muscles adapt to training much less quickly than your cardiovascular system; to stay injury free, you must give them time to catch up.

One piece of equipment you will definitely need is a sport watch with a stopwatch feature. Digital is best; sweep second-hand readings tend to get approximated when you're bouncing along.

Schedule enough time each week to complete the three sessions with rest days in between, rather than trying to squeeze your training into consecutive days. Many people find it helps to start on a weekend. It also helps to pick a running route that's enticing and as free of obstacles—pedestrians and cars—as possible. Think of running an out-and-back route, and at the halfway point, head home.

Try to stick with your plan and avoid missing your scheduled training sessions. If you do have to miss a session, don't try to make up for it by doing double time on your next outing, as this drastically increases the risk of injury. Consistent training works best.

Sherry

Sherry has run numerous marathons, including the Boston Marathon, and even completed an "ironman" competition. But this hasn't always been the lifestyle of the 40-year-old Detroit native. She was a cheerleader throughout high school and refused to do much more than lift a few light weights whenever her friends in college dragged her to the YMCA.

But once Sherry was nearing 30, she started to find it increasingly difficult to fight the extra pounds. Before her pending marriage to her extremely fit and trim fiancé, she decided to take the plunge and bought her first pair of runners since high school. She told herself she would run 15 minutes, 3 days a week, and diet like crazy in the months leading up to her wedding. She was seriously committed to fitting into her size 8 wedding dress.

As the weeks passed, Sherry stuck with her running routine and slimmed down to her desired size. She was surprised at how much she had grown to love the freedom and lightness she felt on her runs. Even her friends commented on her endless good cheer and optimistic attitude. Although she wasn't a negative person before, she had definitely had some mood swings. So when her friend Suzy suggested she join her in training for a half marathon, Sherry didn't hesitate. Ten years later, Sherry is more than hooked on running. She says it's the best part of her day.

Coaching Advice
and the Programs

ARE YOU READY? IT'S TIME TO BELLY UP TO THE LINE AND
put to work everything you've learned so far about distance running. The two c's, commitment and consistency, are the key ingredients. It's only when you take on too much, go too fast, or miss a
large number of training sessions that your workouts go from pleasant to not so pleasant. This chapter outlines the principal framework for the 26-week training programs, including coaching advice
specific to each training phase, and provides some final tips and
goal-setting strategies to help you successfully cross your finish line.

Starting a Marathon and Half-marathon Program
in a Perfect World

Ideally, you will have been running three times a week for the past
year. If it's the half marathon you want to complete, you will have
finished a 10-kilometer (6.2-mile) event, and if you're training for a
full marathon, you will have already run a half marathon.

If this describes your current level of training, you will likely find
the first several weeks of the half- or full-marathon programs outlined in this chapter too easy. If this is the case, review your program

of choice and decide where you are most comfortable starting. The easiest way to figure out where you should start your program is to use the long run as your reference point. You want to match your weekly long run with the appropriate long run in your desired training program. If, for example, the longest run of the week is usually about 20 kilometers (12.4 miles) or 2.5 hours, match this with whichever week recommends an equivalent long run.

Starting a Marathon or a Half-marathon Program for True Beginners

If the above paragraph does not describe you, and instead you are a true beginning runner, the 26-week training programs for the half and full marathon are for you. The programs here are for the true beginner.

Common Questions

Should I start with a 10-kilometer event before attempting the half marathon?

Starting with a 10-kilometer event for your short-term goal is a great idea. The half marathon can be your long-term quest in a year or two. If you're looking for a good learn-to-run-10-kilometers program, you might want to refer to *The Beginning Runner's Handbook,* which includes several proven 13-week walk/run programs.

How do I choose what half or full marathon I should enter?

Go on-line and search for information on marathon and half-marathon events in your chosen location and at your preferred time of year. Or ask your local specialty running store for a listing of half- and full-marathon events. You should make sure you have at least 26 weeks to prepare for your race. It's a wise idea to give yourself an extra couple of weeks in the event that you're sidelined by illness or injury or require some extra time to build endurance and strength.

How will my training progress throughout the 26-week program?

Both the half-and full-marathon programs are carefully designed to include three training sessions: one "short" day, one "short-medium" day, and one "longer" day each week. The programs support the principle that the longer run is the most important element of your training program. As the weeks progress, your long run gets longer every other week. The programs are comprised of an alternating pattern of building and recovery weeks, designed to gradually improve your strength and endurance to prepare your body and mind for the demands of the distance event. A building week essentially means an increase in the intensity and volume of your workouts, whereas the recovery week is less demanding and designed to give your body time to adapt to the increased stresses from the previous week.

Is there a pattern to my training program?

During the third week, we have suggested Saturday or Sunday as your long-workout day, and it follows a 2-week pattern of increased volume followed by a recovery week. Remember, you will be gradually training to cover

The shuffle

- As crazy as it sounds, do the first minute of the running interval **on the spot.** It becomes clear how the run is truly meant to be a shuffle.

- The shuffle technique: upright body carriage, a short swing of the arms, and little steps with no knee lift. You are not bouncing. It is a shuffle. Think of how a boxer looks running in training, or even a dancer doing the cha-cha!

- Your weight should be distributed on the mid- to forefoot, unlike in walking, which is clearly a heel-toe action.

- Remember, the goal is to eventually mesh the walking with the shuffle-jog, so that the body and mind hardly note the difference. The speed is irrelevant: you are learning to run. The speed will come later.

the distance. You will need to measure the distance of your weekend sessions in order to be certain that you are covering the suggested distance in the program.

What is a "shuffle," and why do I have to do it? Why can I not just run right away?

Running is a high-impact sport, which makes it very demanding on the body. The impact of running must be absorbed by all of your muscles, joints, ligaments, and tendons. It takes your body a long time to adjust to these demands. You'll remember that the goal is to keep you healthy and to gradually, through a process of incremental increases in running, build the strength and stamina to complete your goal distance. To avoid injury, you need to build up your running pace very gradually. In the initial stages of your program you want to be moving very slowly in order to be comfortable— the pace can be described as a "shuffle." It is a pace that is similar to a fast walk during which you can easily maintain a conversation. If you cannot maintain a conversation at the shuffle pace, you are going too fast and need to back off.

Will I be expected to have the strength and know-how to run in the first week of training?

No, you are not expected to be able to run right away. Remember, whether you're training for the marathon or half marathon, you will be doing a combination of walking and shuffling for the entire 26-week program.

How does the walking and running combination work?

You will notice that the two midweek sessions consist of timed portions of walking and running. It would be helpful to have a sport watch so that you can keep track of the time. The progressions are designed in such a way that as the walk portions alternate with the shuffle or jog portions, over the next many weeks you will gradually progress to jog timed sections of 10 minutes, 15 minutes, 20 minutes, and on up to 30 minutes. The whole idea is that the walking meshes with the jogging so that your body and mind hardly notice the difference.

Warming up is important. Note that the times shown do not include your warm-up and cool-down times; for those, we suggest a minimum of 5 minutes at the end of each workout. Be sure to allow extra time in your schedule for these essential components. Please note that the distances and estimated times found in your program are just that—estimates, based on a walk/run time of approximately 15 minute miles. In other words, we are suggesting that the average time it will take a beginning distance runner to walk/run 1 mile is 15 minutes. You will have to go by how you feel, which is why we encourage you to measure a route to be certain that you are covering the suggested distance. Some of you will go slower than 15 minutes per mile, and that's fine; others will take significantly less time. Just remember that it depends on the individual, and you just need to be concerned about maintaining a comfortable pace for you. Don't worry about the length of time it takes you to cover your distance.

The run portion of the training should be a very slow jog, more like a shuffle. The pace should be slow so that it almost feels effortless. In fact, it might feel as if you could walk as fast as you are running. If the run is not always at a comfortable "talking" pace, then please slow down!

What is the difference between the half- and full-marathon programs?

The midweek walk/jog sessions, whether on Tuesday and Thursday or Monday and Wednesday, are exactly the same. The only difference between those and the weekend (Saturday or Sunday) long-run day is that the distances indicated are adjusted to correspond to whether you are training for the half or the full marathon.

What are the training programs like?

We've divided the 26-week programs into six 4-week phases and one final 2-week phase. Take each manageable block of training one at a time, and try to stay focused on the workouts, on the advice within each of the workouts, and on the advice within each phase. Don't get too far ahead of yourself. By focusing only on one specific day's scheduled workout, you're less likely to get overwhelmed.

What do I do if I feel I'm not ready to advance to the next week's training schedule?

The best personal monitor is to make sure you are honestly and consistently using your logbook. Regularly record how you felt each day of training; for example, "I completed my Saturday run and felt great," or "I managed to get through the workout, but my hamstring was really bothering me from the halfway mark." Be sure to include lifestyle concerns such as being out late, stressful times at work, sick kids, or whatever else might interfere with optimum training conditions. Trust your instincts—if your recent logbook entries indicate you've been having various difficulties (perhaps a cold, or a nagging pain) it may not be the best time to progress; instead, repeat the same week's training. Remember, everyone progresses differently, so be sure to build a few extra weeks into your training schedule to allow for repeating certain weeks if you need a little extra time to build up strength and endurance before progressing to the next week's challenges.

If you find you have an ache or pain, refer to chapter 9 for detailed information on rating your pain and how to know when you should take a few days' rest. Or, if you catch a cold or flu bug when training and wonder how sick you need to be before taking a day off, refer to chapter 9 for information on what to do if you're sick. Finally, if you do need to take a break of 1 or even 3 weeks, refer to the section at the end of that chapter for guidelines on how to best resume your training program.

Why do the programs increase the length of the long run only every second week? Why don't we just run a little farther each week?

Our training programs use what's called the "overload principle," where each training phase alternates between building and recovery weeks. The objective is to systematically and conservatively overload the body in order to build strength. Although you need to stress the body to prepare it for the demands of the marathon or half marathon, you don't want to be in a continual state of stress, because stress without rest just leads to more stress and in turn to fatigue, burnout, and eventually injury.

I've decided to start with the half marathon, but how do I find a race?

In 26 weeks this beginner program will take you to the half-marathon finish line as safely and comfortably as possible. Find a race that interests you, either by visiting a local specialty running store or by going on-line to find an event farther afield that interests you. Many runners choose a "destination" event so that they can enjoy some well-deserved downtime after such a huge task as completing a half marathon. Or maybe you could think about doing your half marathon with a charity in mind and asking your friends to pledge some dollars for every kilometer of your race.

I've decided to go for the full marathon, but can I do it?

This is a big commitment, but it's doable with the right attitude. We would prefer you start with the half-marathon program and progress from there, but we know that people are making the marathon their initial goal, so we have created a beginner program that will take you to the marathon finish line in 26 weeks. But we want you to be cautious—if, at any point in your training, you don't feel ready to move to the next week of the program, we encourage you to repeat the same week until you feel ready to push forward. The 26 weeks are just a guideline. Beginners will be approaching their training with varying levels of fitness and experience. Our generic programs cannot take into account all of the variables contributing to your individual training.

Before You Get Started, Some Last-minute Advice

Under ideal circumstances the progression of this training program will be smooth and uneventful. However, we're not always dealing with ideal circumstances. You have jobs, children, leaking roofs, and grass to cut. Your training progressions are only one of many demanding aspects of your life, unlike professional athletes whose training is their primary focus. For example, when you have a 7:00 AM 10-kilometer training run and your child wakes up at 3:00 AM having wet the bed, you're not entering your workout under optimal circumstances. Your training progress and response to it are modified by events surrounding it. It is impossible to control all of the variables, and emotional ups and downs are inevitable. The key is to recognize this is a healthy and normal part of any training program. Don't be upset or put off. A word of warning: at some point in your training you will likely experience feelings of extreme fatigue, both physically and mentally, which commonly results in some degree of emotional turmoil. In other words, you will likely encounter emotional highs and lows. But don't be overly concerned—it's all part of being a distance runner and nothing a little extra sleep won't cure.

And finally, remember that all runners experience guilt and disappointment. All runners, even beginners, have performance expectations. When a person misses a workout or performs below expectations it is common to experience guilt and emotional lows. What's surprising is that this makes the process more rewarding, not less, because people find out they have more strength than they thought or ever imagined possible.

The Marathon and Half-marathon Programs

The difference between the marathon and half-marathon programs

The programs for the half and full marathon are identical with the exception of the long run. The scheduled long runs for the marathoners are longer distances than those for the half-marathon runners.

Phase 1: Weeks 1–4

A journey of a thousand miles begins with a single step.
—Lao-tzu, Chinese philosopher

Congratulations! You've taken the first few steps in your half- or full-marathon journey.

Goals for phase 1

1. To begin to establish a comfortable "shuffle" pace as your first stage in learning to run for a few minutes at a time

Table 1
Phase 1 Programs

Pattern	Mon.	Tues.	Wed.	Thurs.	Fri.	Sat. Long-Run Day	Sun.
Week 1 We've begun! Comfortable	Off	Warm-up: Shuffle 5 min. Shuffle 1 min. Walk 2 min. Do this 8 times Cool-down: Walk 5 min. Total time: 34 min.	Off	Warm-up: Walk 5 min. Shuffle 1 min. Walk 2 min. Do this 6 times Cool-down: Walk 5 min. Total time: 28 min.	Optional cross-training day	Warm-up: Walk 5 min. Shuffle 1 min. Walk 2 min. **Half Marathon:** Repeat this for 3 mi. or 5 km **Full Marathon:** Repeat this for 3 mi. or 5 km Cool-down: Walk 5 min.	Walk 20–30 min. Optional for good recovery
Week 2 Building	Off	Warm-up: Walk 5 min. Shuffle 2 min. Walk 2 min. Do this 7 times Cool-down: Walk 5 min. Total time: 38 min.	Off	Warm-up: Walk 5 min. Shuffle 1 min. Walk 2 min. Do this 7 times Cool-down: Walk 5 min. Total time: 31 min.	Cross training	Warm-up: Walk 5 min. Shuffle 1 min. Walk 2 min. **Half Marathon:** Repeat this for 4 mi. or 6.5 km **Full Marathon:** Repeat this for 4 mi. or 6.5 km Cool-down: Walk 5 min.	Walk 20–30 min.
Week 3 Building	Off	Warm-up: Walk 5 min. Shuffle 3 min. Walk 2 min. Do this 7 times Cool-down: Walk 5 min. Total time: 45 min.	Off	Warm-up: Walk 5 min. Shuffle 2 min. Walk 2 min. Do this 6 times Cool-down: Walk 5 min. Total time: 34 min.	Cross training	Warm-up: Walk 5 min. Shuffle 2 min. Walk 2 min. **Half Marathon:** Repeat this for 5 mi. or 8 km **Full Marathon:** Repeat this for 5 mi. or 8 km Cool-down: Walk 5 min.	Walk 20–30 min.
Week 4 Recovery	Off	Warm-up: Walk 5 min. Shuffle 3 min. Walk 2 min. Do this 6 times Cool-down: Walk 5 min. Total 40 min.	Off	Warm-up: Walk 5 min. Shuffle 2 min. Walk 2 min. Do this 5 times Cool-down: Walk 5 min. Total time: 30 min.	Cross training	Warm-up: Walk 5 min. Shuffle 2 min. Walk 2 min. **Half Marathon:** Repeat this for 3 mi. or 5 km **Full Marathon:** Repeat this for 4 mi. or 6.5 km Cool-down: Walk 5 min.	Walk 20–30 min.

2. To confirm your commitment to this new exercise program and to make your three weekly training sessions a priority in your busy life

How you might feel during this phase

With luck, you're feeling excited about your new challenge. It's understandable if you feel some uncertainty, especially during the first few training sessions. Rest assured that before long these feelings will be replaced with a comfortable confidence.

Coaching tips: Find a comfortable shuffle

Most people, at least initially, try too hard and do too much too soon. If you find things too easy to start with, that's good! As your workout time increases, you will find it challenging enough. Here are a few things to consider when you're trying to find your own running pace:

- Both of the walking and jogging portions should be completed at a "talking pace," which means exactly that: you should be able to comfortably carry on a conversation at all times, whether you are walking or jogging. If you find yourself short of breath, you need to slow down.
- The run, or jog, portion of each session is more like a "shuffle-jog." You want it to feel as though you could walk as fast as you run.
- It may sound a little odd, but if you're unsure of how the shuffle should feel, try doing the first minute of your running interval shuffling on the spot. This will give you a clear sense of the slow and easy nature of running at your own pace.

- The long-term goal is for your shuffle-jog and your walk to eventually blend together into continuous jogging. But for the duration of your half- or full-marathon program, there is a clear distinction between jogging and walking.

- In addition to finding a pace that works for you, it's also important in the early stages to establish a solid training pattern. This means you need to decide when, where, and at what time you will do the bulk of your training.

- Make an appointment with yourself, just as you do for the other parts of your life, and do not cancel these new appointments. By making your sessions a priority from the start, you are more likely to stick with your training.

- As the program indicates, spread your sessions evenly over the week: for example, Tuesday, Thursday and Saturday, with optional cross training sessions on Friday and Sunday. For information on cross training, refer to chapter 7.

- You will soon figure out whether you prefer to exercise early in the morning, during your lunchtime break, or at the end of the day. You will find your commitment to the program easier if you establish a weekly pattern for your training times.

Let the important people in your life know you have made this commitment to train for the half or full marathon. Share your excitement, and give them a "heads-up" when you plan to work out, so that they can support you. The time commitment is huge, and there

i **Tips from an elite athlete: Find good footwear**

Two-time Olympic marathoner Bruce Deacon knows all about the importance of good footwear. "The most important equipment you need right now is a pair of good, supportive running shoes. If you haven't already done so, do yourself a favor and head to your nearest specialty running store, with at least 30 to 40 minutes to allow yourself time to be fitted properly. Bring in your old footwear so that the experts can analyze your tread and at the same time look at your gait and foot type. The athletic-footwear world has become very specialized, with shoes to accommodate things like a neutral foot (if that's you, you're lucky), overpronation, supination, you name it, and most companies offer width sizing as well. Do treat yourself and buy the best shoes you can afford. You won't regret it, because you'll be more comfortable and have less chance of injury."

is no doubt it will affect their lives as well as your own. They will respect you for your hard work, and who knows, maybe even join you!

Phase 2: Weeks 5–8

To climb steep hills requires a slow pace at first.
—Shakespeare, *King Henry the Eighth*

Patience is key. Avoid focusing on the work ahead. Instead, feel good about your progress. Each workout brings increased confidence and positive reinforcement: you can do this!

Goals for phase 2

1. To be able to jog consistently for 6 minutes at the end of week 8
2. To truly start to find your own jogging rhythm

How you might feel during this phase

The initial feelings of excitement from your new goal are likely being overshadowed by fatigue and the odd ache or pain. You may be feeling some soreness in muscles you didn't even know you had. These are normal feelings, but you still need to take care of yourself. Now is the time to establish healthy habits such as proper nutrition and hydration, as well as making sure you have adequate sleep.

Coaching tips: Find your own personal jogging rhythm

Your goal is to become physically comfortable while learning to run. This means finding an easy, relaxed rhythm that you naturally settle into each time you

Table 2
Phase 2 Programs

Pattern	Mon.	Tues.	Wed.	Thurs.	Fri.	Sat. Long-Run Day	Sun.
Week 5 Building. Okay, no more shuffling; you're jogging now!	Off	Warm-up: Walk 5 min. Jog 3 min. Walk 1 min. Do this 9 times. Cool-down: Walk 5 min. Total time: 46 min.	Off	Warm-up: Walk 5 min. Jog 2 min. Walk 1 min. Do this 8 times. Cool-down: Walk 5 min. Total time: 34 min.	Cross training	Warm-up: Walk 5 min. Jog 2 min. Walk 1 min. **Half Marathon:** Repeat this for 4 mi. or 6.5 km. **Full Marathon:** Repeat this for 5 mi. or 8 km. Cool-down: Walk 5 min.	Walk 20–30 min.
Week 6 Building	Off	Warm-up: Walk 5 min. Jog 5 min. Walk 1 min. Do this 7 times. Cool-down: Walk 5 min. Total time: 52 min.	Off	Warm-up: Walk 5 min. Jog 3 min. Walk 1 min. Do this 7 times. Cool-down: Walk 5 min. Total time: 38 min.	Cross training	Warm-up: Walk 5 min. Jog 3 min. Walk 1 min. **Half Marathon:** Repeat this for 5 mi. or 8 km. **Full Marathon:** Repeat this for 6 mi. or 10 km. Cool-down: Walk 5 min.	Walk 20–30 min.
Week 7 Building	Off	Warm-up: Walk 5 min. Jog 6 min. Walk 1 min. Do this 6 times. Cool-down: Walk 5 min. Total time: 52 min.	Off	Warm-up: Walk 5 min. Jog 4 min. Walk 1 min. Do this 6 times. Cool-down: Walk 5 min. Total time: 40 min.	Cross training	Warm-up: Walk 5 min. Jog 4 min. Walk 1 min. **Half Marathon:** Repeat this for 6 mi. or 10 km. **Full Marathon:** Repeat this for 8 mi. or 13 km. Cool-down: Walk 5 min.	Walk 20–30 min.
Week 8 Recovery	Off	Warm-up: Walk 5 min. Jog 4 min. Walk 1 min. Do this 6 times. Cool-down: Walk 5 min. Total time: 40 min.	Off	Warm-up: Walk 5 min. Jog 2 min. Walk 1 min. Do this 10 times. Cool-down: Walk 5 min. Total time: 40 min.	Cross training	Warm-up: Walk 5 min. Jog 2 min. Walk 1 min. **Half Marathon:** Repeat this for 4 mi. or 6.5 km. **Full Marathon:** Repeat this for 6 mi. or 10 km. Cool-down: Walk 5 min.	Walk 20–30 min.

walk/jog. Try incorporating the following suggestions on your next training run:

- Pace is definitely part of finding a comfortable running rhythm. You should be able to carry on a conversation at all times. If you're out of breath, you need to slow down.
- As the jog portion increases, remember it's your arm action that will help you to maintain your rhythm and pace.
- Try to keep your shoulders square and relaxed and your arm action quick, and ensure your elbows are tucked close to your sides.
- Distance running is all about efficiency and conserving energy, which means shorter strides, with very little knee lift.
- In addition to your rhythm, think about your technique. Keep your body upright, keep your arms relaxed and close to your body, and take small steps, without a strong knee lift.
- When you're running, try to remember this is a shuffle and avoid bouncing. Your weight should be distributed on the mid- to forefoot, unlike in walking, which is a heel-toe action.

You've penciled in your commitment to training, but it's essential to keep an actual training logbook. It might be in your daytimer, or the calendar in your kitchen, or it might be a separate bedside book you write in each night. Jot down the time of day of your session, how you felt mentally and physically, and anything going on in your life that may have affected you, such as a late night at work or a stressful situation at home. It's helpful to be able to look back and track how you've been handling the program, both as a confidence builder and as a way to prevent injury.

Phase 3: Weeks 9–12

> *The Two Rules of Perseverance:*
> *Rule #1: Take one more step.*
> *Rule #2: When you don't think you can take one more step, refer to Rule #1.*
> —H. Jackson Brown Jr., American author

Persevere and stay on track with your training. Each completed session brings you that much closer to achieving your goal.

Goals for phase 3

1. To be able to jog continuously for 10 minutes
2. To understand the importance of the non-running elements of your training

How you might feel during this phase

The volume of the workload has increased, and although it's a positive lifestyle change, you might be surprised at the far-reaching impact it has on the other areas of your life. Work, sleep, nutrition, and family are all affected. Adjustments and shifts in lifestyle take time. Persevere, and have faith that it will all fall into place as it should.

Table 3
Phase 3 Programs

Pattern	Mon.	Tues.	Wed.	Thurs.	Fri.	Sat. Long-Run Day	Sun.
Week 9 Building	Off	Warm-up: Walk 5 min. Jog 6 min. Walk 1 min. Do this 7 times Cool-down: Walk 5 min. Total time: 59 min.	Off	Warm-up: Walk 5 min. Jog 4 min. Walk 1 min. Do this 6 times Cool-down: Walk 5 min. Total time: 40 min.	Cross training	Warm-up: Walk 5 min. Jog 4 min. Walk 1 min. **Half Marathon:** Repeat this for 5 mi. or 8 km **Full Marathon:** Repeat this for 9 mi. or 14.5 km Cool-down: Walk 5 min.	Walk 20–30 min.
Week 10 Moderate, recovery	Off	Warm-up: Walk 5 min. Jog 8 min. Walk 1 min. Do this 4 times Cool-down: Walk 5 min. Total time: 46 min.	Off	Warm-up: Walk 5 min. Jog 5 min. Walk 1 min. Do this 5 times Cool-down: Walk 5 min. Total time: 40 min.	Cross training	Warm-up: Walk 5 min. Jog 5 min. Walk 1 min. **Half Marathon:** Repeat this for 4 mi. or 6.5 km **Full Marathon:** Repeat this for 7 mi. or 11 km Cool-down: Walk 5 min.	Walk 20–30 min.
Week 11 Building	Off	Warm-up: Walk 5 min. Jog 10 min. Walk 1 min. Do this 4 times Cool-down: Walk 5 min. Total time: 54 min.	Off	Warm-up: Walk 5 min. Jog 6 min. Walk 1 min. Do this 5 times Cool-down: Walk 5 min. Total time: 45 min.	Cross training	Warm-up: Walk 5 min. Jog 6 min. Walk 1 min. **Half Marathon:** Repeat this for 6 mi. or 10 km **Full Marathon:** Repeat this for 10 mi. or 16 km Cool-down: Walk 5 min.	Walk 20–30 min.
Week 12 Easy, recovery	Off	Warm-up: Walk 5 min. Jog 8 min. Walk 1 min. Do this 3 times Cool-down: Walk 5 min. Total time: 37 min.	Off	Warm-up: Walk 5 min. Jog 5 min. Walk 1 min. Do this 4 times Cool-down: Walk 5 min. Total time: 34 min.	Cross training	Warm-up: Walk 5 min. Jog 5 min. Walk 1 min. **Half Marathon:** Repeat this for 5 mi. or 8 km **Full Marathon:** Repeat this for 8 mi. or 13 km Cool-down: Walk 5 min.	Walk 20–30 min.

Coaching tips: Put the non-running pieces of your puzzle in place

It's simply not enough to complete your three workout sessions each week. You need to create a positive framework that supports your goals. Here are some tips to remain healthy, rested, and upbeat throughout the 26 weeks of your training:

- Look forward to your recovery weeks. The decreased workload and volume will give you the mental boost and confidence to tackle the increases during the building weeks.

- Try to incorporate a cross-training day into your workout pattern. Besides being relaxing and fun, cross training provides you with the opportunity to improve core strength that will help prevent injuries as your body adjusts to the impact of running and walking.

- A relaxed Sunday walk is a great way to recover from your weekly long run on Saturday. Walking keeps the circulation flowing and helps your legs to recover.

- Make sure you work on your flexibility. Walking and running shortens the tendons and muscles, especially in your calves and hamstrings. Stretching before and after your workouts will ensure better recovery and help to prevent injury.

- Measure the distance of your runs. You will notice in the training program that we have included suggested times as well as specific distances in both kilometers and miles. Take a drive, and measure some of your running routes by using the car's odometer.

Measuring the length of your longer training runs will give you a sense of how long it will take you to complete the various distances. Also, running a measured route gives you confidence that you are getting closer to completing your distance.

- Body awareness is important. Pay attention to any small aches and pains. Keep track of them in your logbook to ensure they are only a result of working hard and disappear as the body gets stronger. It will take a while for you to grow accustomed to some increased fatigue as well as slight aches or pains from training.

- If you miss a week or two of training, do your best to gradually resume the program. Avoid jumping back into the schedule where you left off. Rushing drastically increases the chances of injuring yourself.

Phase 4: Weeks 13–16

You *have to stay in shape. My grandmother, she started walking 5 miles a day when she was 60. She's 97 today and we don't know where the hell she is.*
—Ellen DeGeneres, American comedian

Milestone: You are over halfway through the program: Congratulations!

Goals for phase 4

1. To comfortably and safely walk/run half the distance of your event. For the marathoners that means a half marathon, or 13.1 miles (21 kilometers). For the half marathoners it means about 6.5 miles (10.5 kilometers) or jumping into a 10-kilometer event to test yourself.

Table 4
Phase 4 Programs

Pattern	Mon.	Tues.	Wed.	Thurs.	Fri.	Sat. Long-Run Day	Sun.
Week 13 Building	Off	Warm-up: Walk 5 min. Jog 10 min. Walk 1 min. Do this 4 times. Cool-down: Walk 5 min. Total time: 54 min.	Off	Warm-up: Walk 5 min. Jog 3 min. Walk 1 min. Do this 3 times. Cool-down: Walk 5 min. Total time: 37 min.	Cross training	Warm-up: Walk 5 min. Jog 8 min. Walk 1 min. **Half Marathon:** Repeat this for 6 mi. or 10 km. **Full Marathon:** Repeat this for 11 mi. or 18 km. Cool-down: Walk 5 min.	Walk 20–30 min.
Week 14 Moderate, recovery	Off	Warm-up: Walk 5 min. Jog 15 min. Walk 1 min. Do this 2 times. Cool-down: Walk 5 min. Total time: 42 min.	Off	Warm-up: Walk 5 min. Jog 10 min. Walk 1 min. Do this 3 times. Cool-down: Walk 5 min. Total time: 43 min.	Cross training	Warm-up: Walk 5 min. Jog 10 min. Walk 1 min. **Half Marathon:** Repeat this for 5 mi. or 8 km. **Full Marathon:** Repeat this for 9 mi. or 14.5 km. Cool-down: Walk 5 min.	Walk 20–30 min.
Week 15 Building	Off	Warm-up: Walk 5 min. Jog 15 min. Walk 1 min. Do this 3 times. Cool-down: Walk 5 min. Total time: 58 min.	Off	Warm-up: Walk 5 min. Jog 10 min. Walk 1 min. Do this 3 times. Cool-down: Walk 5 min. Total time: 43 min.	Cross training	Warm-up: Walk 5 min. Jog 10 min. Walk 1 min. **Half Marathon:** Repeat this for 6 mi. or 10 km or a 10-km event. **Full Marathon:** Repeat this for 13 mi. or 21 km or a half-marathon event. Cool-down: Walk 5 min.	Walk 20–30 min.
Week 16 Easy, recovery	Off	Warm-up: Walk 5 min. Jog 15 min. Walk 1 min. Do this 2 times. Cool-down: Walk 5 min. Total time: 42 min.	Off	Warm-up: Walk 5 min. Jog 10 min. Walk 1 min. Do this 2 times. Cool-down: Walk 5 min. Total time: 32 min.	Cross training	Warm-up: Walk 5 min. Jog 10 min. Walk 1 min. **Half Marathon:** Repeat this for 4 mi. or 6.5 km. **Full Marathon:** Repeat this for 8 mi. or 13 km. Cool-down: Walk 5 min.	Walk 20–30 min.

How you might feel during this phase

It's normal to feel a little anxious before your 10-kilometer or half-marathon event. After all, this might be the first race of your life. Refer to the section later in this chapter on preparing for event day. Reviewing this section will alleviate some of the pressure you're feeling. And remember, some anxiety can actually help your performance!

Coaching tips: Tackle the hills along your routes

Including hills in your training runs is a great way to build stamina needed to complete the half-marathon distance. If there are hills on either your half- or full-marathon course, it's even more important to include at least a few hills on your regular training routes. If you decide to ease back and walk up the hills on race day, that's okay. And even if your course doesn't have any hills, you still might want to consider including some in the odd workout to build strength. Even some courses that don't have big hills have inclines that can be ominous during the event... it's always good to practice on some rolling terrain.

How to run hills

- Lean slightly into the hill while hinging at the waist.
- Keep the stomach and back strong.
- Focus your attention only a few feet in front of you.
- Shorten the leg stride slightly with small, quick steps.

- The most common mistake people make is over-striding up a hill. Test it yourself: try one hill with small, quick steps and the next with a longer stride. Guaranteed, you will discover your effort is greater with the longer stride.

- Land on the balls of the feet, and the second one foot touches the ground, consciously lift the other knee as quickly as possible and a little higher than normal.

- Remember to pump your arms. As always, the arms dictate the pace.

- Be patient. Take it one step at a time, and before you know it you will be going down the other side. Regardless of whether you walk or run up hills, getting to the top is a great confidence booster.

Tips

- Remember to take care of yourself. Make your daily habits as optimal as possible: healthy, balanced meals; good hydration; lots of rest, and keep stress levels at a minimum. At this stage your body is your temple. You want to do all you can to feel your very best.

- Be honest with yourself. If you're not feeling confident and are not comfortable progressing as the program advances, it's likely you've not been able to establish a consistent pattern of training each week. Maybe you haven't been able to complete all of your weekly sessions, for a variety of reasons. If you're unable to do your homework and complete at least the minimum of three walk/run sessions each week, you may need longer to realistically pursue your goal of safely and comfortably completing a half or full marathon. There's nothing wrong in discovering that your program needs some minor adjusting. You may need to give yourself 36, 46, or even 56 weeks to prepare for your distance-running goal. Remember, these are only guidelines that we have laid out for you—it's up to you to figure out what is required for your fitness level.

Congratulations: you're over halfway through your program! You deserve a treat of some kind for yourself, something that allows you to reinforce your sense of accomplishment. For some of you it may mean a nice brunch or dinner. For others, you may feel a quiet celebration is what you need such as walking on the beach or in the woods or taking a long, hot bath. Do something that inspires you and makes you feel great, whatever that may be.

Phase 5: Weeks 17–20

Some people think that successful people are born that way. A champion is someone who has fallen off the horse a dozen times and gotten back on the horse a dozen times. Successful people never give up.

—Jean Driscoll, eight-time Boston Marathon winner (wheelchair division), five-time Paralympic gold medalist (track-and-field)

This is a difficult time in the program. Remember your long-term goal, and keep in mind how far you have come!

Goals for phase 5

1. To build your continual running time to approximately 20 or 30 minutes
2. To establish a strong mental attitude regarding your running

Table 5
Phase 5 Programs

Pattern	Mon.	Tues.	Wed.	Thurs.	Fri.	Sat. Long-Run Day	Sun.
Week 17 Building	Off	Warm-up: Walk 5 min. Jog 20 min. Walk 1 min. Do this 2 times. Cool-down: Walk 5 min. Total time: 52 min.	Off	Warm-up: Walk 5 min. Jog 15 min. Walk 1 min. Do this 2 times. Cool-down: Walk 5 min. Total time: 42 min.	Cross training	Warm-up: Walk 5 min. Jog 15 min. Walk 1 min. **Half Marathon:** Repeat this for 8 mi. or 13 km. **Full Marathon:** Repeat this for 14 mi. or 22.5 km. Cool-down: Walk 5 min.	Walk 20–30 min.
Week 18 Moderate, recovery	Off	Warm-up: Walk 5 min. Jog 20 min. Walk 1 min. Cool-down: Walk 5 min. Total time: 31 min.	Off	Warm-up: Walk 5 min. Jog 15 min. Walk 1 min. Do this 2 times. Cool-down: Walk 5 min. Total time: 42 min.	Cross training	Warm-up: Walk 5 min. Jog 15 min. Walk 1 min. **Half Marathon:** Repeat this for 5 mi. or 8 km. **Full Marathon:** Repeat this for 10 mi. or 16 km. Cool-down: Walk 5 min.	Walk 20–30 min.
Week 19 Building	Off	Warm-up: Walk 5 min. Jog 20 min. Walk 1 min. Do this 2 times. Cool-down: Walk 5 min. Total time: 52 min.	Off	Warm-up: Walk 5 min. Jog 15 min. Walk 1 min. Do this 2 times. Cool-down: Walk 5 min. Total time: 42 min.	Cross training	Warm-up: Walk 5 min. Jog 15 min. Walk 1 min. **Half Marathon:** Repeat this for 9 mi. or 14.5 km. **Full Marathon:** Repeat this for 16 mi. or 25.5 km. Cool-down: Walk 5 min.	Walk 20–30 min.
Week 20 Easy, recovery	Off	Warm-up: Walk 5 min. Jog 30 min. Cool-down: Walk 5 min. Total time: 40 min.	Off	Warm-up: Walk 5 min. Jog 10 min. Walk 1 min. Do this 2 times. Cool-down: Walk 5 min. Total time: 32 min.	Cross training	Warm-up: Walk 5 min. Jog 10 min. Walk 1 min. **Half Marathon:** Repeat this for 4 mi. or 6.5 km. **Full Marathon:** Repeat this for 8 mi. or 13 km. Cool-down: Walk 5 min.	Walk 20–30 min.

How you might feel during this phase

At this point in your training, you will soon, if you haven't already, experience the far-reaching effects of physical fatigue. It's common to have days, or hours, when you are happy one moment and sad the next. The roller coaster of emotions is, in large part, directly proportional to your level of fatigue. If you can, try to get some extra sleep, and make sure you include some downtime in your week. Reading, or watching a movie with your family, is just what you need right now.

Coaching tips: Create the mental strength to run continuously

This is the most demanding training phase in your program. For many of you, it will be the hardest you have ever pushed yourself, both mentally and physically. This is when you begin to understand the psychological demands of distance training. Whether it's during a demanding training run or in the hours leading up to your weekly long run, it's sometimes difficult to be positive and optimistic. Training your mind for the demands of your event is as important as training your body. The following are a few tools to help you to mentally prepare yourself for the rigors of distance running:

- Seek out company. Find someone to join you, especially for your long weekend sessions. Have him or her follow you on a bike, roller blades, or drive ahead in a car to encourage you at various spots along your route. Just knowing you have support along the way helps you to overcome the emotional lows and self-doubt that are characteristic of long training runs and harder midweek sessions. It's also a great motivator, and it can be a fun way to include your friends in your experience.

- If you haven't already, find someone who has direct experience training for, and completing, a distance event. Ask your mentor questions about training, pre-race jitters, or any running questions you might be pondering. This kind of support is great for bolstering confidence. Knowing that others have gone before you and accomplished your dream is motivational. It often prompts a beginning runner to think, "If they can do this, why can't I?"

- Take a break from the pavement or asphalt. Vary the terrain, and try to find some grass or trails. It will help prevent unnecessary aches or pains to give the body a break from the impact of harder surfaces. It's motivating to find a new place to run, like a park or trail system you've never been to before.

- Water running is great, especially if you're experiencing sore muscles or extreme fatigue. Pool or water running can be strength-building as well as therapeutic. Turn to chapter 7 for a detailed description of pool running.

Phase 6: Weeks 21–24

The body does not want to do this. As you run, it tells you to stop, but the mind must be strong. It is the will to succeed.

—Jacqueline Gareau, Canadian 1980 Boston Marathon champion

Physically you are working through the sessions, but it's the strength in your mind that is the driving force. Keep up the good work!

Goals for phase 6

1. To begin preparing yourself for completing your distance event by completing an event-day dress rehearsal
2. To be physically and mentally successful at completing the two longest training sessions in your program

How you might feel during this phase

You may have a few aches and pains and some general fatigue. However, you are enjoying your increased confidence, and you now see yourself as a distance runner.

Coaching tips: Complete your event-day dress rehearsal

We have gradually increased your peak mileage in weeks 21 and 23. Over the next 4 weeks, you will reach the maximum mileage needed in your preparation to safely and comfortably complete your event distance. In an

Table 6
Phase 6 Programs

Pattern	Mon.	Tues.	Wed.	Thurs.	Fri.	Sat. Long Run Day	Sun.
Week 21 Building, working on mileage preparation	Off	Warm-up: Walk 5 min. Jog 30 min. Cool-down: Walk 5 min. Total time: 40 min.	Off	Warm-up: Walk 5 min. Jog 20 min. Cool-down: Walk 5 min. Total time: 30 min.	Cross training	Warm-up: Walk 5 min. Jog 20 min. Walk 1 min. **Half Marathon:** Repeat this for 9 mi. or 14.5 km. **Full Marathon:** Repeat this for 18 mi. or 29 km. Cool-down: Walk 5 min.	Walk 20–30 min.
Week 22 Recovery	Off	Warm-up: Walk 5 min. Jog 15 min. Walk 1 min. Do this 2 times. Cool-down: Walk 5 min. Total time: 42 min.	Off	Warm-up: Walk 5 min. Jog 30 min. Cool-down: Walk 5 min. Total time: 40 min.	Cross training	Warm-up: Walk 5 min. Jog 30 min. Walk 1 min. **Half Marathon:** Repeat this for 5 mi. or 8 km. **Full Marathon:** Repeat this for 10 mi. or 16 km. (Event practice! Set up water stations at approx. distances of those found at the event.) Cool-down: Walk 5 min.	Walk 20–30 min.
Week 23 Peak mileage	Off	Warm-up: Walk 5 min. Jog 30 min. Cool-down: Walk 5 min. Total time: 40 min.	Off	Warm-up: Walk 5 min. Jog 20 min. Cool-down: Walk 5 min. Total time: 30 min.	Cross training	Warm-up: Walk 5 min. Jog 20 min. Walk 1 min. **Half Marathon:** Repeat this for 11 mi. or 18 km. **Full Marathon:** Repeat this for 20 mi. or 32 km. Cool-down: Walk 5 min.	Walk 20–30 min.
Week 24 Moderate, recovery	Off	Warm-up: Walk 5 min. Jog 20 min. Walk 1 min. Do this 2 times. Cool-down: Walk 5 min. Total time: 52 min.	Off	Warm-up: Walk 5 min. Jog 20 min. Cool-down: Walk 5 min. Total time: 30 min.	Cross training	Warm-up: Walk 5 min. Jog 30 min. Walk 1 min. **Half Marathon:** Repeat this for 8 mi. or 13 km. **Full Marathon:** Repeat this for 16 mi. or 25.5 km. Cool-down: Walk 5 min.	Walk 20–30 min.

- Your event practice session is a good chance for you to practice refueling and rehydrating as you walk. It's a good idea to review the section in this book on hydration and overhydration. You want to take in enough liquid, but it's also dangerous to take in too much.

- Take time to treat yourself. Indulge yourself after your successful long session each week. After all, every building week is a milestone. Celebrate after your long run with a massage, glass of wine, or piece of chocolate cake, and have some fun. Moderation is the key, but at the end of every training week, you deserve a mini-celebration!

effort to mentally prepare you for the big event, we suggest you organize an event-day practice by doing the following:

- Map out a course over 10 miles (16 kilometers), with an "official" start and finish time.

- Imagine yourself on event day, and go through the practice session over 10 miles as though it were race day. Encourage your friends and family members to be there for you at the "start" and maybe along the course and at the finish.

- Refer to the next section in this chapter on race-day preparation, and try to treat this day in a similar manner.

- Do some research on the course you will be completing in a few weeks by reviewing the organizers' Web site. Find out the number of water stations they are planning to set up along the route and the approximate distance between each station.

- Chart out the water stations, which will give you a focus while you jog, just as they will during your event. Try to start with a plan to jog from one station to the next, with your walk breaks at each station. Maintain your focus on running for as long as possible.

- The official event Web site should list what will be provided at the water stations. Some, for example, offer water or sport drinks and occasionally some sort of fuel-replacement bar.

- Try not to feel pressure, and remember that it's only about covering the distance. If you find you need to walk sooner than the water station, take your breaks when necessary.

- To this point in your preparation, you have been alternating jogging stints of 10, 15, 20, and 30 minutes, so you can be relaxed and run for the duration that is most comfortable.
- Sometimes you will go through periods where you feel great and jog for 30 minutes; at other times you may have a stint of running that doesn't feel great, and you would be better off taking a walk break.
- Some of you will take a very methodical approach, sticking to a set amount of running, say 10-, 15-, 20-, or 30-minute stints with a 1-minute walk break. What's important is finding what works best for you. Remember, there is no right or wrong way to approach the finish line.

Phase 7: Weeks 25–26

Every person needs to have their moment in the sun, when they raise their arms in victory, knowing that on this day, at this hour, they were at their very best.
—H. Jackson Brown Jr., American author

You've made it! Only 2 weeks to go before the big event. At this point the hard work is finished. Your final training days are simply fine-tuning. Enjoy yourself, and congratulations.

Goals for phase 7

1. To safely complete your half- or full-marathon event, using whatever walk/run pattern you feel is best for you

Table 7
Phase 7 Programs

Pattern	Mon.	Tues.	Wed.	Thurs.	Fri.	Sat. Long Run Day	Sun.
Week 25 Easy, recovery	Off	Warm-up: Walk 5 min. Jog 30 min. Cool-down: Walk 5 min. Total time: 40 min.	Off	Warm-up: Walk 5 min. Jog 15 min. Cool-down: Walk 5 min. Total time: 25 min.	Cross training	Warm-up: Walk 5 min. Jog 15 min. Walk 1 min. **Half Marathon:** Repeat this for 4 mi. or 6.5 km. **Full Marathon:** Repeat this for 8 mi. or 13 km. Cool-down: Walk 5 min.	Walk 20–30 min.
Week 26 You did it! Easy, recovery, rest for EVENT DAY!	Off	Warm-up: Walk 5 min. Jog 30 min. Cool-down: Walk 5 min. Total time: 40 min.	Off	Warm-up: Walk 5 min. Jog 20 min. Cool-down: Walk 5 min. Total time: 30 min.	Cross training	EVENT DAY! Remember to warm up: Walk 5 min. Jog 30 min. Walk 1 min. Jog 20 min. Walk 1 min. Jog 15 min. Walk 1 min. Choose combinations, or toss the watch and run/walk as you feel for the HALF/FULL MARATHON!	Walk 20–30 min. Congrats!

How you might feel during this phase

Race day is looming, and it's likely you're feeling anxious and possibly a little nervous. Try to focus on enjoying your last few workouts and the extra time you have off from training. This is your taper period where your workouts are shorter and less demanding.

Coaching tips: Don't change anything just before race day

Good planning includes not just good training, but putting all the pieces in place: physical and mental well-being, nutrition, hydration, and equipment. In the last 2 weeks before your event, it's not a good idea to introduce anything new to your training or your diet. To help you prepare for race day, review the following commonly asked questions for all of the last-minute advice you will need for a great marathon or half-marathon day.

Common Questions

How do I mentally prepare myself for my event?

During your last few workouts, visualize yourself on race day, at the start, feeling confident and strong. Think about how you will choose your combinations of 10-, 15-, 20-, or 30-minute stints of running followed by 1 minute of walking. You've done this routine many times before, so it will come naturally on race day. Don't forget imagining your exhilaration as you cross the finish line, with your arms in the air and a smile on your face!

How can I feel more confident for race day?

Review your logbook and reflect upon your experience over the past 26 weeks or so, and recall all that you have learned and accomplished over the course of your training program. You've had 26 weeks of physical and mental preparation and significant lifestyle changes, and you've adjusted to the tremendous demands on your body. In truth, you already know how it is going to feel on race day, and familiarity is a huge part of making your dream a reality. You've established personal patterns that have worked to get you through all the workouts, including learning to run and completing all of your peak mileage sessions. Remind yourself: if you were able to complete all of your long runs before the marathon, you can also do it on race day.

Should I estimate how long it will take to complete my event?

As you progress through your training program and become more confident and comfortable with the run/walk combinations, it can be motivating to monitor your run/walk pace. Use your long-run completion time to estimate your pace per mile or kilometer. If you want to estimate your approximate event finishing time, use the Event-Day Pace Chart on the following page: find your pace per mile or kilometer, and extrapolate the finishing time for a marathon or half marathon. Keep in mind that you're improving and doing more running every week, so your pace will change over the months of training. Also, it's a good idea for beginning distance runners to add 5 to 10 minutes to their

Table 8

Event-Day Pace Chart

Minutes Per Mile	5 km	10 km	20 km	Half Marathon	30 km	40 km	Marathon
7:00	21:45	43:30	1:27:00	1:31:32	2:10:30	2:54:00	3:03:03
7:15	22:30	45:01	1:30:02	1:35:00	2:15:04	3:00:06	3:10:00
7:30	23:18	46:36	1:33:12	1:38:20	2:19:48	3:06:24	3:16:39
7:45	24:04	48:07	1:36:15	1:41:33	2:24:23	3:12:30	3:23:06
8:00	24:51	49:42	1:39:24	1:44:52	2:29:06	3:18:48	3:29:45
8:15	25:37	51:14	1:42:28	1:48:06	2:33:42	3:24:56	3:36:12
8:30	26:24	52:48	1:45:36	1:51:25	2:38:24	3:31:12	3:42:51
8:45	27:10	54:20	1:48:40	1:54:39	2:43:00	3:27:21	3:49:18
9:00	27:57	55:54	1:51:48	1:58:00	2:47:42	3:43:36	3:56:00
9:15	28:43	57:26	1:54:52	2:01:12	2:52:20	3:49:44	4:02:24
9:30	29:30	59:00	1:58:00	2:04:33	2:57:00	3:56:00	4:09:03
9:45	30:16	1:00:32	2:01:06	2:08:21	3:01:39	4:02:24	4:16:42
10:00	31:04	1:02:08	2:04:16	2:11:07	3:06:24	4:08:32	4:22:12
10:15	31:51	1:03:41	2.07.23	2.14.22	3:11:04	4:14:46	4:28:45
10:30	32:36	1:05:12	2:10:24	2:17:34	3:15:36	4:20:48	4:35:08
10:45	33:24	1:06:48	2:13:36	2:20:56	3:20:24	4:27:11	4:41:51
11:00	34:09	1:08:18	2:16:36	2:24:12	3:24:55	4:33:13	4:48:15
11:15	34:57	1:09:54	2:19:49	2:27:29	3:29:43	4:39:37	4:54:58
11:30	35:44	1:11:28	2:22:55	2:30:45	3:34:22	4:45:50	5:01:31
11:45	36:30	1:13:01	2:26:01	2:34:02	3:39:02	4:52:03	5:08:04
12:00	37:15	1:14:30	2:29:02	2:37:14	3:43:33	4:58:04	5:14:29
12:15	38:04	1:16:07	2:32:14	2:40:35	3:48:21	5:04:28	5:21:11
12:30	38:50	1:17:40	2:35:21	2:43:52	3:53:01	5:10:41	5:27:44
12:45	39:37	1:19:13	2:38:27	2:47:09	3:57:41	5:16:54	5:34:17
13:00	40:23	1:20:47	2:41:33	2:50:25	4:02:20	5:23:07	5:40:51
13:15	41:10	1:22:20	2:44:40	2:53:42	4:07:00	5:29:20	5:47:24
13:30	41:57	1:23:53	2:47:46	2:56:59	4:11:39	5:35:32	5:53:57
13:45	42:43	1:25:26	2:50:53	3:00:15	4:16:19	5:41:45	6:00:30
14:00	43:30	1:27:00	2:53:59	3:03:32	4:20:59	5:47:58	6:07:04
14:15	44:16	1:28:33	2:57:05	3:06:49	4:25:38	5:54:11	6:13:37
14:30	45:03	1:30:06	3:00:12	3:10:05	4:30:18	6:00:24	6:20:10
14:45	45:50	1:31:39	3:03:18	3:13:22	4:34:57	6:06:37	6:26:44
15:00	46:36	1:33:12	3:06:25	3:16:38	4:39:37	6:12:49	6:33:17

estimated half-marathon finishing time and 10 to 15 minutes to their approximate marathon finishing time.

Is it important to know my pace?

The specific pace, whether it's 10-minute miles or 12-minute miles, is not important, but it is useful information for several reasons. If you know your running pace, it will help you to stay relaxed and avoid the common mistake of starting your race too fast, which can often result in problems later in an event. Also, establishing your long-run pace enables you to estimate the finishing time of your long runs and these 2-, 3-, and sometimes 4-hour runs so that you are better able to organize the other areas of your life.

What are some other reasons for knowing my pace time?

Establishing an approximate finishing time for your event will give your support people an idea of where you will be at different points on the course. This information will also allow you to plan your transportation and post-race festivities.

Fueling the Athlete

Meal planning does not take time away from your training—it is part of your training.
—Dallas Parsons, registered sport dietitian

MARATHON RUNNERS GET HUNGRY. THEY NEED FOOD—A lot of it. But not just any food will fuel you to the finish line. Optimal nutrition and hydration are key players in enhancing your athletic performance. A car won't go without the proper fuel in its tank; nor will your body.

Marathon running places significant demands on your body. If you ignore your body's need for proper fuel, you will put yourself at increased risk for fatigue, injury, and illness. By giving your diet the attention it deserves, your training sessions will be more productive, your recovery time will be shorter, and, most importantly, you will feel better.

The Runner's Training Diet

The three keys to healthy eating are balance, variety, and moderation. A fourth key can be added in these times of highly processed

So, what's a serving?

The following would constitute an average serving: a slice (20 grams) of bread, a cup (250 milliliters) of cereal, a banana, a potato, ¾ cup of cooked beans, 2 eggs or 3 ounces (90 grams) of cooked meat, which is about the same size as a pack of playing cards.

1 serving of grains

¾ cup oatmeal

1 cup shredded wheat

1 slice high-fiber bread

½ cup cooked brown rice

1 serving of fruits and veggies

1 cup raw spinach

1 cup cooked broccoli

1 cup baby carrots

1 pear

1 cup berries

Meat and alternatives

5 oz. cooked salmon

3 oz. cooked chicken

1½ cups lentil soup

3½ oz. tofu

¾ cup black beans

Milk or soy

1 cup fat-free milk

1 cup low-fat soy beverage

¾ cup low-fat yogurt

2 oz. reduced-fat cheese

"fast foods"—namely, that food should be as close to natural as possible.

Balance is about eating from all the main food categories, including fruits, vegetables, grains, meat alternatives, meat, and dairy products—with exceptions, of course, for those who choose to follow a form of vegetarian diet. Remember that no one food group can provide you with all the nutrients you need. A slab of steak with a few peas on the side is not a balanced meal; nor is pasta every day for a month, supplemented by the occasional trip to the salad bar.

Variety means choosing a selection of foods from each main food group every day to ensure a healthy diet. No single food, no matter how nutritious, should dominate your diet or even your intake from one group. Oranges, for example, provide a lot of vitamin C, but eating oranges to the exclusion of other wonderful fruits such as apples, pears, melons, and bananas—each of which has different nutritional strengths—will not result in optimum health.

Moderation ensures that you eat neither too much nor too little. Dietitians suggest at least four servings of grain products and seven servings of fruits and vegetables every day. If milk products are part of your diet, dietitians suggest at least two servings of them per day (three to four for adolescents and pregnant or nursing women). As well, each person should eat two servings of meat or alternative sources of protein (for example, tofu or baked beans) per day.

"Natural foods" might conjure up images of health food stores, but the phrase really just means foods that either are not processed or are processed as little as possible. Such foods tend to be better for you, because they generally contain more nutrients and fewer additives (such as fats) than foods that have been more heavily processed. For example, potatoes are better for you than potato chips, bread made from whole wheat flour is better than bread made from enriched white flour, and apples are better than apple juice. This is not to say that junk food must never pass your lips, just that it should play a minor role in your diet.

What about Fluids?

When it comes to distance runners, water is just as important as food. Vancouver sport dietitian Dallas Parsons suggests, "Dehydration is a leading cause of early onset fatigue. All athletes need to drink enough fluids to replace sweat losses and to maintain optimal fluid balance."

You lose water all the time through perspiration, respiration, and excretion. When you exercise, your body heats up, and in turn you sweat more.

How much water is enough?

Recently, overhydration has become an issue of concern. However, it's still safe to say that the majority of people don't drink enough water, especially when there is the added demand of marathon or half-marathon training programs.

Experts recommend that sedentary folks take in 6 to 8 glasses of fluids each day. As the intensity and duration of your exercise increase, so do your fluid requirements.

Daily hydration strategies from dietitian Dallas Parsons

- Watch TV with a glass of water beside you, and take a sip during commercials.
- Keep a water bottle or tall glass of water at your desk.
- Stash a full water bottle in the car and in your workout bag.
- Drink a small glass of water before or with meals.
- Ask for water along with alcoholic or caffeinated drinks you order.
- Start your day with a glass of cool water.
- Order sparkling water with a squeeze of lemon at business lunches.

It's also important to factor in the temperature around you and the clothing or equipment you're wearing. A couple of hours before your run, try to drink 2 glasses of water, and drink another glass 15 minutes before heading out the door. Distance runners need to stay hydrated on their long runs by taking in water every 30 minutes while running and then drinking 2 to 3 glasses within 10 to 20 minutes after ending the run. Remember, these are just guidelines; a good way to know if you are properly hydrated after intense exercise is to weigh yourself before and after. Weight loss during exercise represents water loss you did not replace during your run.

People new to distance running may experience leg cramps. This could be the result of dehydration, low serum sodium levels (low salt in the blood), or the training as muscles adapt to longer distances. Try to stay hydrated, and make sure you're getting enough salt in your diet.

It takes time for your body to adjust to taking in fluids before and during a training session. Don't leave this part of your planning to the last minute. Make sure you drink before your training sessions, and remember to stay hydrated during your long runs by carrying a water bottle with you.

Sport drinks

There are many different kinds of sport drinks on the market. Check the back of the bottle for a list of ingredients. Many replace electrolytes such as salt and potassium; others provide carbohydrates that are needed for distance runners. And some drinks will replace both electrolytes and carbohydrates. You should consider using a sport drink during your longer runs—they often provide the boost of energy your body needs in the later stages of a 2- or 3-hour workout.

Some marathoners prefer to carry their own water bottle, which is usually a bottle fastened to a waist belt. It might take some time to become accustomed to the feel of a water bottle carrier, so plan ahead and wear it on some of your training runs.

What about overhydration?

One of the problems with the growing number of athletes who are taking a run/walk approach to the marathon is the increasing rate of hyponatremia, or overhydration. As University of British Columbia sport medicine physician Dr. Jack Taunton points out, "The big concern that we are starting to see in marathoners who are walking large portions of the event is overhydration. Basically, these folks are walking through the aid stations, ingesting too much water, and end up with hyponatremia. It can be and has been fatal."

Hyponatremia is a shortage of sodium in the blood. This state occurs when runners sweat excessively, lose too much salt, and drink excessive amounts of water, which then dilutes the blood's sodium content even more.

Signs of overhydration

- Dizziness
- Headache
- Confusion
- Fainting
- Fatigue
- Weakness
- Cramping
- Nausea
- Vomiting
- Bloating and puffiness in the face and fingers
- Loss of consciousness
- Fluid in the lungs
- Seizures
- Coma
- In severe cases, death

Why has overhydration become such a concern?

"There is an obsession that people have in this current society with drinking fluids and being concerned about dehydration. Everyone seems to have a water bottle on their desk or with them at all times," says Dr. Taunton. He finds at least part of the reason for our concerns in sport medicine, and in the American College of Sport Medicine guidelines, which became increasingly aggressive in terms of encouraging people to drink more and more fluids. Now we're starting to see marathon organizers taking two and three aid stations out of the races in order to reduce the risk of people taking in too much fluid.

For beginning runners, hyponatremia is a significant concern, but it's not a problem for the very fast. When elite runners are running fast, their gastrointestinal systems' absorption rate is impaired. This means "it is virtually impossible for those finishing a marathon in under 3 hours to take in too much water," says Dr. Taunton. However, when people are moving at a shuffle pace, they haven't shunted the blood supply away from the gut to the exercising muscle. Your body still has the capability of absorbing a great percentage of the water you drink, so you end up increasing your total blood volume and diluting your sodium sources. This is when you run into problems. This is why it's essential for beginners to play close attention to their fluid intake and remember to alternate water with electrolyte solutions along the way.

To avoid overhydration, consume an average of 4 to 8 oz. (120 to 240 milliliters) of sport drink every 15 to

30 minutes during your race. You may want to increase your salt intake slightly 2 or 3 days before the race; sprinkle a little salt on your food once or twice a day, hydrate with a sport drink the day before, and enjoy cereals and breads as part of your carbohydrate-loading plan.

Getting Your Nutrients

Vitamins and minerals

Regardless of whether you're a vegan, eat organic food regularly, or knock back a sirloin every few days, your cells are looking for some key nutrients to do their job. The human body uses carbohydrates, protein, and fat from food to fuel itself, and in order for the metabolic processes to work properly, it requires vitamins and minerals. Here are a few tips on vitamins from Parsons:

- You will need fewer vitamin and mineral supplements if you have a balanced diet and take in an adequate amount of calories.
- Milk, egg yolks, and vegetables are a good source of vitamin A.
- Many fruits and vegetables provide vitamins B and C.
- Meat, whole grains, leafy vegetables, soybeans, poultry, and fish offer B vitamins.
- Vitamin D is found in egg yolks, fish oils, canned sardines, fortified milk, and soy-milk products.
- Wheat germ, sunflower oil, and whole grain cereals have vitamin E.
- Vitamin K is found in vegetables, especially in green, leafy ones.
- Calcium is found in dairy products, fortified soy products, fortified orange juice, almonds, and oranges.

- Meat and alternatives, enriched cereals, clams, and lentils offer iron.

Runners need carbohydrates

If you're a distance runner, you need a fair amount of carbohydrates in your diet. Different from proteins and fat, carbohydrates are quick and easy to break down and offer an almost immediate source of fuel. Extra glucose can also be stored in your muscles and liver as glycogen, the main source of fuel for muscle movement. Human beings have a low capacity for storing glycogen, which is why you need to replace it daily.

The Glycemic Index (GI) was originally developed for people with diabetes; it classifies carbohydrate-containing foods by how much they raise blood sugar levels compared with a standard food. A food with a high GI raises blood sugar levels more quickly than a moderate or low glycemic food. Eating foods with a low GI may help to provide lasting energy for long runs and control your appetite.

The main difficulty with using the GI is that the index value remains true only if the food is eaten in isolation, but this is not practical, because food is mostly eaten in mixed meals. Dietitians say this doesn't mean the GI has no value, just that it is a complex approach. What is most important is that, as a runner, you choose quality food sources of carbohydrates such as whole grains, fruits, and vegetables to fuel your body.

Allow time to digest food. Approximate digestion times: 1–2 hours for carbohydrates, 2–4 hours for protein, 4–6 hours for fats.

Protein

Dallas Parsons encourages runners to include protein in their diets: "Although carbohydrates are the main staple of a runner's diet, protein is also very important for the growth, maintenance, and repair of muscles and other tissues." Protein is needed for the formation of hemoglobin, which carries oxygen to working muscles and provides support for the immune system. Protein also slows digestion and increases people's satisfaction levels after finishing meals. The best choices for protein sources include lean red meats, fish and seafood, poultry, beans and lentils, tofu, eggs, and low-fat dairy or soy products. Aim to include one of these foods in each main meal.

Good and bad fat

We have all read about the hazards of too much fat, but too little fat or none at all is also bad. The best or healthiest sources include omega-3 fatty acids. These are essential nutrients that help your body to function properly. Salmon, tuna, flaxseed oil, canola oil, soybean oil, fortified eggs, and dairy products are just a few of the options for including omega-3 fatty acids in your diet. Other healthy fat choices include olives, nuts, seeds, vegetable oil, and avocado.

One serving of fat equals 1 teaspoon of oil. Try to limit your amount of added fats to three to six servings per day.

Bad fats such as trans-fatty acids should be avoided or consumed only on rare occasions. Trans-fatty acids

Aim to choose these sources of carbohydrates most often

- Grains such as brown rice, quinoa, amaranth, kasha, and wild rice
- Whole and sprouted wheat bread and whole wheat pasta
- High-fiber and whole grain cereal
- Brightly colored fruits and vegetables
- Dark-green and leafy vegetables

are commonly found in highly processed food products, including some margarines, and usually in fast foods and snack foods as well as in commercially baked cookies, muffins, and cakes. Look at the "Nutrition Facts" label and aim to get as close as possible to "0 trans fats."

The vegetarian runner

Being a vegetarian means different things to different people. Some vegetarians eat fish and chicken; others abstain from all animal products, including dairy products. Regardless of the type of vegetarian you are, the basic principles of healthy eating remain. Remember, it's all about a well-rounded, wholesome diet that remains flexible to allow a moderate amount of "treats." Vegetarians who don't eat any seafood or meat can easily miss out on some vitamins and minerals that are difficult to find in a strict vegetarian diet. These nutrients include protein, calcium, iron, zinc, vitamin B_{12}, and vitamin D. Fortified foods such as breakfast cereals, textured soy products, and soy beverages provide many of these key nutrients. A multivitamin and mineral supplement would also be a worthwhile investment. Alternative protein sources such as tofu, beans, lentils, nuts, seeds, soy beverages, and meat analogues provide adequate protein when eaten in the correct amounts.

If you are unsure whether you are meeting all your energy and nutrient requirements, or if you need additional supplementation, consult a registered dietitian. If you are experiencing unusual fatigue, you should make an appointment to see your physician to have your iron stores (ferritin) checked.

Daily Meal Planning and Calorie Levels

Now that you have read about the nutrients your body needs to be well fueled for running, your next questions might be: how do I get all this good nutrition in and how much do I need? It may sound more complicated than it is. Says Dallas Parsons, your daily energy requirement (caloric needs) is determined by four main factors: resting metabolic rate, thermal effect of food, daily activity, and purposeful exercise. As a runner, 55 to 60 percent of your calories should come from carbohydrates, 15 to 20 percent from protein, and the remaining 20 to 25 percent from fat. Despite all the numbers and serving recommendations, there is no prescription diet that meets everyone's needs. Always adapt recommendations to your personal preferences and requirements.

 Insights into smart meal planning for runners

- These are essential kitchen tools for a busy athlete: indoor grill, steamer, and slow cooker.
- Make a 1 week meal plan. Figure out how many dinners and lunches you need. Think about your training and whether you need anything special, such as sport-drink powder.
- Buy a small chalkboard for the kitchen and use it for a running list of foods that need to be replenished.
- Keep your kitchen well stocked with foods that are handy in a pinch, such as frozen meats, breads and vegetables, canned beans, tomato sauce, pasta, and dried fruit.
- Go shopping every week for fresh fruits and vegetables.
- Make double the recipe and freeze leftovers, or take them for lunch.
- Scout out some simple recipes. Ask your running mates for their favorite quick recipe.
- Pack lunches, snacks, training food, and fluids the night before.
- Keep a food journal to ensure you are eating a complete and adequate diet. Reflect on your entries for clues on how to improve your eating habits.

Estimating your daily calorie needs

Calories

30–32 cal/kg (2.2 lb.) body weight per day on rest days

33–38 cal/kg body weight per day on 1-hour running days

39–43 cal/kg body weight per day on 2-hour running days

44–50 cal/kg body weight per day on 3-hour running days

Carbohydrates

4–5 g/kg/day on recovery days

5–6 g/kg/day for 1 hour of running

7–8 g/kg/day for 2 hours of running

8–9 g/kg/day for 3 hours of running

Protein

1.0–1.2 g/kg/day for an adult runner to maintain mass

1.2–1.4 g/kg/day for an adult runner building muscle mass

Note: 2.0 g/kg/day is the maximum usable amount of protein for adults.

Fat

Minimum 1.0 g/kg/day for an adult runner, depending on energy needs

Table 9
Food-Group Servings Based on Calorie Level

Food Group	Number of Servings for		
	2,000 cal	2,500 cal	3,000 cal
Grains	6	8	10
Fruits and vegetables	2 fruit, 4 veg	3 fruit, 4 veg	4 fruit, 5 veg
Milk and soy products	2–3	2–3	3
Meat and alternatives	2	2–3	3
Fats	3	3–4	4

The Basics of Eating for Training and Competition

Before running, why should I eat?

Eating before running has three functions: to top up muscle, liver, and glycogen stores; to ensure adequate blood sugar levels; and to prevent hunger before and during exercise.

What runners eat is just as important as why they eat

Try to choose lower-fiber, carbohydrate-rich foods such as breads, grains, cereals, fruits, and vegetables. Include small amounts of protein. If, for example, you eat 2 to 4 hours before you run, sources of protein might include 2 ounces (56 grams) of lean meat, 2 table-spoons (30 milliliters) of peanut butter, ¾ cup (180 milliliters) of low-fat yogurt, 1 cup (250 milliliters) of milk or ½ cup (125 milliliters) of cottage cheese, and 1 egg. Avoid high-fat foods. On race day, eat only familiar foods. Try out your pre-race meal during training to ensure that it agrees with your stomach. If you suffer from a nervous stomach and have difficulty eating before races, try a liquid meal such as a fruit smoothie or a meal-replacement drink. Your pre-running meal should be low in fat, low in fiber, and high in carbohydrates. And remember to show up to training well hydrated. Drink 2 cups (500 milliliters) of fluid 2 hours before.

How much should I eat?

Sport dietitian Dallas Parsons says pre-workout food choices vary widely among runners. The best advice is to experiment during training. This will help you find a pre-race meal that works for you. If you are racing out of town, be sure to plan your pre-race meal. Ask yourself: what will I eat, when will I eat it, and where will I get it?

Use the guidelines in table 10 to start.

Table 10

Time between Exercise and Meal	Carbohydrates	Calories	Example for 65 kg (143 lb.) Runner
15 minutes*	25 g	100	1 energy gel with water
1 hour prior	1 g carb/kg body weight	250	65 g carb = 1 bagel (30 g), 2 tsp jam (10 g), 1 banana (27 g)
2 hours prior	2 g carb/kg body weight	400–600	130 g carb = 1 cup fruit yogurt (45 g), 1 cup cooked oatmeal (30 g), 1.5 tbsp brown sugar (25 g), 8 oz orange juice (30 g)
3 hours prior	3 g carb/kg body weight	700–900	195 g carb = 2 cups pasta (80 g), 1 cup lean meat and tomato sauce (40 g), 2 slices bread (40 g), ½ cups cranberry cocktail (45 g)

*Only if tried in practice; this is a typical interval for many endurance athletes

Marathon and Half Marathon

Is it okay to eat sugar before I exercise?

Some runners are concerned that they may experience a drop in blood sugar levels and energy if they eat carbohydrates in the hour prior to exercise. Research shows that although an increase in plasma insulin following carbohydrate ingestion in the hour prior to exercise can result in temporary low blood sugars during subsequent exercise, there is no convincing evidence that this is always associated with impaired running performance. With that said, individual practice should be based on individual experience.

If this is a concern, avoid eating simple sugars (for example, candy, gels, sport drinks) 30 to 45 minutes before training. The night before your race, eat a mixed meal that includes carbohydrates, protein, and vegetables. Here are some examples:

- pasta with tomato-vegetable sauce, shrimp, chicken, or lean ground meat
- tofu and vegetable stir-fry over rice or noodles
- bean-and-vegetable soup with salad, bread, and milk
- grilled fish, steamed vegetables, and brown rice

If eating 2 or more hours before running, eat a small high-carbohydrate meal that is low in fat and has a minor amount of protein for lasting energy. For example:

- low-fat yogurt, with low-fat granola with raisins
- bagel with peanut butter and honey and juice
- ready-to-eat cold cereal with low-fat, flavored soy milk
- oatmeal with 1 percent milk and a piece of fruit

Best foods for recovery

During training or races, your body loses fluids and uses a lot of muscle glycogen. Carbohydrates and water are what your body needs to replenish. If you're dehydrated and glycogen-depleted, your body cannot recover and perform well during subsequent training. As part of your training, make it a habit to drink at least 2 cups (500 milliliters) of fluids as soon as you can after finishing a run. Ideally, refuel 10 to 15 minutes post-exercise.

- pita pocket with vegetables and tuna, grapes, and arrowroot cookies
- chicken breast with rice, steamed vegetables, and fruit yogurt

If eating 1 hour before running, drink a liquid meal such as a yogurt-and-fruit smoothie or meal-replacement drink. Sport bars are another alternative, but be sure to choose one that provides at least 30 grams (1 ounce) of carbohydrate and less than 10 grams of protein. Consider the following options:

- bagel, jam, milk
- fruit smoothie made with milk, yogurt, juice, and fruit
- toast with peanut butter and honey, sport drink
- pasta with tomato sauce, milk

If running first thing in the morning, have a glass of sport drink, diluted fruit juice, or water, and an energy gel. These options will provide approximately 75 to 100 calories and should prevent light-headedness or low blood sugars during a 30- to 45-minute run, provided a good meal was eaten the night before.

Fuel for your long runs

Sport dietitian Dallas Parsons says:

- If you are well fueled before you run and training for only 1 hour, water will suffice in most cases.
- If the weather is very hot, or if you are unaccustomed to warm temperatures, a sport drink is a good idea even for shorter runs, because it encourages drinking and replenishment of fluids,

carbohydrates, and sodium. For training runs lasting longer than 2 hours, take along a carbohydrate source to keep up your energy supply to your working muscles and brain. Start with 30 grams of carbohydrate per hour after the first hour. Some people need more than this and may go up to 60 grams per hour.

- Another general guideline for fueling while running is 1 gram of carbohydrate per kilogram of body weight per hour after the first hour. Energy gels and sport drinks are among the most popular supplements used during long runs. Some runners can tolerate solids, such as bites of a sport energy bar or Fig Newton cookies.

By race day you should have a plan that combines the best fluid and fuel replacement to support your needs and preferences. On the day, you may experience unexpected conditions such as wind, hot weather, or cramping; you should be ready and able to adjust your nutrition plan as needed.

Be sure to replenish your fluids after running. Weight lost during running is due to loss of water. For every pound (half kilogram) of weight lost during a workout, drink 3 cups (750 milliliters) of fluid.

After interval work or long training runs, which put more stress on your muscles and energy stores, it's important to rehydrate and have a recovery snack within 30 minutes of completing exercise. Blood flow to the muscles is greater then, and muscle cells are more insulin-sensitive. At this time the body is able to maximize glycogen replenishment and muscle repair.

Read the labels on your sport products

You may be wondering whether you need to use special sport products such as protein powders, meal-replacement drinks, and energy bars. Aside from being expensive, these products can quickly add excess calories to your day. Read the labels carefully to check their energy, carbohydrate, protein, and fat content, and always consume with plenty of water. If choosing a bar, look for one with a three- or four-to-one ratio of carb to protein and less than 3 grams of fat per 100 calories.

To prevent unwanted weight gain, yet maximize your recovery, avoid adding extra calories to your day to meet your recovery needs. Instead, rearrange your daily snacks or meals to accommodate a post-run snack.

In addition to carbohydrates, include some protein to aid repair of muscle tissues. Some examples of good post-workout snacks are:

- Flavored yogurt and fruit
- Dried fruit and some nuts
- Flavored milk and a banana
- Peanut-butter-and-honey sandwich
- Fruit juice and soy nuts
- Cereal and milk
- Sport drink and bagel
- Sport energy bar and fruit

Simple Nutrition Tips

- If you are experiencing more cravings for sweets than usual, try adding some protein to your snacks, such as low-fat yogurt with a few tablespoons of cereal, or almonds and an apple.
- Drinking full-strength juice within 30 minutes before running may contribute to side stitches or abdominal cramps. If you need some liquid calories, try diluting juice with an equal amount of water or drinking a sport drink.
- A skim-milk latte is a great way to celebrate a long run with your partners, satisfy your caffeine fix, and boost your recovery. Order a water to go with it.

Runner's diarrhea is an embarrassing and frustrating condition that can really put a damper on long runs.

If you suffer from this, these hints may help:

- Run hydrated. Try drinking 1½ cups (350 milliliters) of water 1½ to 2 hours before you run.
- Drink a quarter cup of fluid (two or three gulps) every 15 minutes during your long runs.
- Don't eat within an hour of running. You may even need to give yourself 2 hours to digest food.
- Eat low-fiber foods such as breakfast cereals (less than 3 grams of fiber per serving), English muffin and jelly, pretzels, saltines, flavored yogurt, or pancakes with syrup.

A multivitamin and mineral supplement daily is a good idea for most runners. If you think you need additional supplements, talk to a registered dietitian or physician. Choose a high-quality, reputable brand, and look for one that provides a little extra iron and calcium.

If you're feeling unusually tired during workouts, you may be dehydrated. Try stepping up your fluid intakes, and monitor your urine output. You should empty a full bladder of clear or pale-yellow urine every 2 to 3 hours.

Are there foods I should avoid before running?

Yes, but individual tolerances must be considered. Foods that tend to cause problems for runners include spicy seasonings, full-strength fruit juice, whole grain breads (more than 4 grams of fiber per slice), high-fiber cereals (more than 6 grams of fiber per 30 grams), prunes, figs, cabbage, broccoli, onions, nuts, beans, candy, or high-fat snack foods.

The Mental Side
of the Marathon

DIAL IT IN; FOCUS; DIG DEEP. THESE ARE JUST A FEW expressions used to motivate us to reach within ourselves and discover our full potential. For the marathon runner, often the mental barriers are the greatest obstacles to overcome. As with most things in life, whether it's your career, education, or personal relationships, achievement in distance running does not come easily.

Early in your training program, you will realize that a fit body won't travel far if there isn't a fit mind traveling along with it. Sometime during your training—probably on a cold, rainy, windswept day—you may find yourself staring out the window and discover that you have a remarkable capacity for making excuses. At this point, you will understand the adage that marathon training is as much mental as it is physical.

Staying on track with any kind of fitness program is a challenge for most of us. But the ability to stay focused and motivated for the duration of a 6-month training program is a huge challenge. Your body and mind will benefit, but the action of run/walking itself will be laborious even for the most motivated individuals. There are bound to be days or even weeks when you just don't feel like running. It's important to know that all athletes dip in motivation; you are not alone in this. Everyone gets tired, and everyone has other areas of life that can interfere with training. This chapter offers clear strategies and practical suggestions on how to push through those difficult days and overcome the mental roadblocks, waning motivation, and nagging uncertainty familiar to most distance runners.

Seeing Yourself as a Runner

Before you can learn about the mental side of distance running, you must believe you can become a distance runner. Seeing yourself in a new way is not easy, especially if you have not been involved in sports in the past or if you've gained some weight over the years and feel you are some way away from feeling like your old, sporty self. To this point we have talked only about how, with the right training and a graduated approach such as the distance-running programs in this book, you can make it to the start line of a half or full marathon. However, training and completing one of these events is an amazing goal. For many of you, this might be the most difficult undertaking you have ever attempted. You want to become a runner and may even dream about it, but actually seeing yourself going from a sedentary person to someone who is up in the morning and walk/running for 45 minutes is another story. How do people do it? How do people change their patterns and lifestyles? Others have done it, and so can you.

How to change old habits

You've heard it before: couch potato turns marathon runner; a pack-a-day smoker climbs Mount Kilimanjaro. Some people change old habits with seemingly little effort, whereas others talk about the same troubles for weeks, months, or even years but are still stuck in the same insufferable spot.

Everyone has one or two—or three—maddening inclinations that we call bad habits. Whether it's merely a foible familiar only to family and friends or a more serious pattern like smoking or overeating, change is not easy. You have only to check the shelves of your local bookstore to recognize that changing patterns is an industry in itself. Besides "self-help" books and videos with the principal goal of helping people achieve the life they desire, there is also an increasing demand for hands-on courses and training programs.

Research on changing behaviors

American social science researchers J.O. Prochaska and C.C. DiClemente created the "transtheoretical" model of change. The model, originally conceptualized for problem behaviors such as alcohol abuse, supports the belief that change is made through a process of small, incremental adjustments. Central to the transtheoretical model are its five stages of change, which describe how people alter a problem behavior or acquire a positive routine. The theory suggests that everyone travels through several common stages when they are attempting to change a pattern or behavior.

Stages of change

1. *Pre-contemplation:* At this time there is little or no desire for change. A person may not even recognize that there is a problem. For example, someone at this stage could be content with walking to work as daily exercise, and, although he passes runners on his walk, he is not interested in beginning any sort of running regime.

2. *Contemplation:* At this stage people are aware of a problem and are giving serious consideration to change. In other words, they have started to take responsibility for the habit or pattern. For example, our walker in stage 1 above may have been told by his doctor that he needs to develop a healthier lifestyle that includes aerobic exercise. He continues to walk to work and finds himself wondering what it might be like to join one of the runners that breeze by him.

3. *Preparation:* This is the point at which individuals are getting ready to take action. They have decided to address a problem, and they are taking concrete steps toward that goal. Our walker has been fitted for running shoes and has bought other gear. He has talked to a friend who also wants to begin running.

4. *Action:* During this stage people are altering behavior and environment in order to tackle their problem. They are taking action. The individual and his friend sign up and attend a local running clinic for beginners.

5. *Maintenance:* Now people are working to avoid slipping back into their old patterns. Significant

changes have been made; our friend and his partner have been running regularly three times a week and have developed a schedule that works for both of them. But there may still be some longing for the old days and former habits.

Belief in oneself

When a person decides to become a marathon runner and thus puts the stages-of-change model to the test, it's important to believe in one's ability to effectively control specific events in one's life, which is an important component of changing behaviors. Researchers and mental health counselors think this belief is what separates people who change successfully from those who remain in chronic contemplation mode. Research supports belief in the power of positive thinking; it suggests that confident people generally have optimistic thoughts about being able to cope with a large variety of stressors. In contrast, people who have difficulty in believing in themselves are more prone to depression, anxiety, and helplessness. These individuals often have low self-esteem and hold pessimistic thoughts about their accomplishments and personal development.

Cheerleading from friends and family is great, but improving one's belief in oneself requires action. A strong belief in your ability to overcome problem situations needs more than positive self-talk. Building that belief is a slow and gradual process of experiencing and *acknowledging* accomplishments. As a result of incorporating incremental changes, people are more likely to experience success and ultimately achieve their goals.

Unfortunately, a common problem in building confidence is taking on too much, too soon. The result is often feelings of failure or, worse, reversion to old habits.

Believing in oneself has a strong correlation to successful change. If we are confident in our ability to change, we generally will succeed. For example, studies show that people who think they are the most creative turn out to be the most creative. For most of us, confidence is something built over time by way of small, incremental accomplishments. These accomplishments are the building blocks that make the foundation of our system of belief in ourselves.

The importance of small and timely changes

Experiencing small successes is key to moving through the stages of change. Failure to change usually occurs when people attempt to change too quickly or before they have committed themselves to a systematic and sequential plan. This can be damaging, as it reinforces low confidence and the belief that one cannot or will not change. Others may have intervened at the incorrect stage—for example, a running coach may have distributed a workout schedule without realizing that not everyone in the room was at the same stage of change.

The dangers of negative feedback

Evidence indicates that humans are most sensitive and responsive to the negative. You have only to watch the television news to realize that disaster stories are far better at drawing our attention than feel-good stories.

Based on this reasoning, the stages-of-change model incorporates numerous processes to teach readiness skills that slowly and gradually guide individuals through each of the five stages of change.

The model indicates that during the process of change, negative feedback more easily undermines one's confidence than encouragement builds it. Self-doubt can often lead to not trying or to tentative efforts that quickly and easily confirm negative self-evaluation. For example, when a beginning exerciser starts an overly aggressive running program without a strong support system, he or she rarely experiences success. Feelings of failure arise when the lone runner is forced to walk parts of a 20-minute run. If that same person joins a friend or running group and uses a slow, gradual, walk/run approach, he or she has a greater likelihood of experiencing feelings of success. And don't forget to acknowledge the small and large achievements along your marathon pathway. Acknowledgment of your achievements solidifies your success and in turn helps to formalize in your mind the idea that you are improving. All of these elements are part of the process of building confidence and inner strength.

The challenge to change is a daunting process for even the most strong willed. As we have learned, willpower alone is not enough to shift our patterns. In order to rid ourselves of a habit, we need a systematic and sequential plan that provides us with the opportunity to experience success and in turn build our self-confidence. For people who want to complete a half or full marathon, it all begins not with poetry but prose:

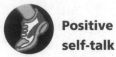

Positive self-talk

- Congratulate yourself. After a good run, or even a so-so run, stop and think about how good you feel at having completed your running goal for the day. Remember the feeling of accomplishment, so that the next time you lack motivation to get out the door for your run, you can remind yourself with confidence that exercise makes you feel good!

- Talk to yourself. Remind yourself that the farther you go in the training process, the easier it gets. There is always a reason not to exercise, but the reasons to exercise are almost always better. As your fitness increases, so will your self-esteem and confidence. Both are key to making it through the training program and to the marathon finish line.

- Think positively. Focus on what feels good, not on what hurts. At the beginning of your marathon program, you are bound to experience various aches and pains that develop as your body begins to adapt to the new stress levels. This is especially true for your long run. Be patient; this is all part of the longer process of becoming a distance runner.

one foot in front of the other. One step and then one stride.

Train your mind for the marathon

"The amount of physical training required to complete a half or full marathon is substantial. The time commitment required to prepare and ultimately compete is perhaps not fully understood until you're actually living it! Then there is the challenge of your mental training—when your mind and thoughts wander during actual runs," says Vancouver sport psychologist Dr. Whitney Sedgwick.

Adults have the ability to mentally "multitask," which can be both efficient and distracting. When running, you may find your thoughts jumping from topic to topic. This isn't necessarily a bad thing. It would not be realistic to attempt to focus only on your running technique, muscle aches, the course you're running, your competitors, et cetera, during a run. In fact, some runners separate themselves from these types of thoughts in order to distract themselves. There are accounts of runners mentally building a house and decorating every room in their mind while running. Others have conducted lengthy, detailed conversations in their mind in order to pass the time of the run. Most runners combine the strategies, sometimes thinking about bodily sensations, at other times separating themselves mentally from the event. So, recognize that maintaining a continuous focus is difficult and may not be sustainable, particularly for longer distances.

The importance of what you say to yourself is crucial to effective performance, as is having a plan for mental success.

Finding the motivation

We all know that on some days we're more motivated than on others. Motivation fluctuates and shifts in all areas of life. Some days you feel energized to tackle a list of chores; at other times, lounging around the house seems much more appealing. Dr. Sedgwick, who works with all levels of athletes, points out that within almost any relationship there are moments when you are giving more than you are receiving, and vice versa. She says the same is true for physical training: "As long as we understand that it is almost impossible to be 100 percent motivated to train and compete all of the time, then we can be more realistic in the expectations we put on ourselves." By using some of the tips outlined in this chapter, you can set clear and realistic goals that should keep you highly motivated most of the time.

Kari

Kari is a 40-year-old outreach worker and mother of two. Before moving back to Canada and adopting her twin daughters from Honduras, she was a program officer in Yemen, working toward the joint goal of strengthening and expanding democracy worldwide.

Kari gained valuable experience and, as a girl from a small Canadian mining town, she traveled to places she had only imagined in her dreams. Many of the countries she worked in or visited were politically unstable, and for the most part there were very few opportunities for her to exercise. Fitness facilities were difficult to find, as were safe places to jog or walk. She found herself putting her health on the proverbial back burner.

When her daughters were tiny, she would take them for long walks in the stroller. Once they started to get older, Kari realized that if she wanted to keep up with the lively little girls, she would have to increase her energy level. This would mean losing a little weight and beginning a regular exercise program. She cut down on sweets and started to walk/jog several times a week, a good way to gradually improve her fitness without getting hurt. Eventually, she found her jogging time to be significantly longer than the time she spent walking.

Today, Kari mostly jogs on her own, but occasionally her friend Marcy joins her. Marcy is a sport psychologist and an amazing athlete who was on the swim team in college, and she now jogs to stay fit. Marcy has been trying to persuade Kari to train for an upcoming half marathon in the fall. "Even though I would love to, I have convinced myself that only true athletes like Marcy run marathons, and I'm definitely not an athlete," says Kari. "I've always been smart and good at school, but I was never picked for any of the teams at school."

Marcy is certain Kari can run the half-marathon distance, but her friend has to first see herself as an athlete. Kari has agreed to volunteer as a course marshal at this year's half marathon, and Marcy believes seeing all the different ages, shapes, sizes, and abilities of the participants will be Kari's first step toward viewing herself as an athlete capable of completing a half or even a full marathon.

Running, like all sports, is an opportunity to enjoy pleasure and excitement that are sometimes hard to find. Once we discover a sport that suits us, often passion and meaning come with the ongoing process of overcoming challenges. Whether you're a downhill skier hoping to master a black diamond run or a runner wanting to complete a marathon, the pleasure of anticipation is the same. Regardless of the challenge, in order for an athlete to be motivated to train and compete he or she must find meaning in the endeavor. Without a commitment, there is little motivation to pursue a goal. Training week in and week out over the course of several months is not a task for the weak at heart. The half or full marathon cannot be something you "should" or "have" to complete. Ultimately, to be successful, it needs to be a dream you "want" to fulfill.

Goal Setting

The process of setting goals and planning the best pathway to meet objectives allows men and women to choose where they want to go in life. We all know people who seemingly have it all with very little effort and few clear plans. However, for the most part, people don't achieve on sheer luck; undoubtedly, some behind-the-scenes work has gone on. Though luck might come into it, people's careers, education, and athletic achievements generally involve goal setting.

Goals can provide you with a long-term vision and act as a short-term motivator. For example, if your long-term goal is to complete a marathon in 6 months, it will act as a daily motivator to complete your scheduled run.

Different types of goals

There are various types of goals that are useful in maintaining focus and motivation, including these:

- Time-oriented goals: "I'll run 10 kilometers on Saturday in under 48 minutes"
- Lifestyle goals: "I will get a minimum of 8 hours of sleep nightly"
- Social goals: "I'll train with my friend John on Wednesday after work"
- Process goals—these focus on your ongoing performance and can be physical, psychological, or technical in nature, such as concentrating on your running form during a workout: "Tonight is Fartlek training as part of my speedwork"
- Outcome goals—these are geared toward your anticipated end result: "I plan to finish this race in a new personal best time"

Common goal-setting problems

Goals can be great motivators, but people fall into numerous traps when they don't carefully consider all of the factors associated with their challenge. These traps can often limit effective goal setting and decrease motivation. Common problems include goals that are too vague, overly challenging, or not meaningful to the individual.

The acronym SMARTER can assist you to achieve your goals:

S   for *specific*. Is your goal clear and concise?

M   for *measurable*. Can you determine whether you reached your goal?

A   for *adjustable*. Can the goal be modified if needed?

R   for *realistic*. Is the goal appropriate for you, your level of fitness, resources, et cetera?

T   for *time-based*. Is there a time frame around the goal?

E   for *exciting*. Are you looking forward to achieving the goal?

R   for *recorded*. Have you written down the goal?

Using, for example, the goal of incorporating weight training into your routine, a poorly set goal might be: "I think I'll try to learn about weight training." A SMARTER goal would be: "I will go to the introductory class on weight training at my gym this Monday at 7 PM."

Dr. Sedgwick suggests that a common pitfall for all athletes is negative self-talk. If you catch yourself saying

"I have to..." frequently, it is a good idea to step back and reconnect with your original reasons for running. A person who, in contrast, has a high level of motivation to do a marathon would frequently use positive self-talk such as "I want to train" or "I get to go for a run." Even better, add an exclamation point: "I want to train!" You can see it doesn't take much to give yourself a positive message.

Make Running a Routine

Making running part of your routine increases your chances of sticking with it and achieving your marathon goals. Dr. Sedgwick suggests that when starting a new exercise or running program it's important to, as early as possible, establish habits or routines that work for you. Before you cross the finish line of a half or full marathon, ideally you will have created and maintained a running routine that easily fits into your daily life. Through trial and error you will figure out what works for you. You will learn whether you run better alone or with a group, the best time of day for you to run, and the pre-run diet that works for your body. These are a few examples of tests you will repeat throughout your training until your best options become known and routine. For some people, running will become as much a part of their daily routine as brushing their teeth.

Mix It Up

Beginning marathoners usually start their training with an abundance of excitement and motivation, but maintaining enthusiasm over the months of training isn't

Craig

Craig was never really into running; he preferred sports like hockey and skiing. "I always thought running was for tiny guys. I'm 6 foot 4 and built more like a football player than the waifs I see running marathons." But when Craig's good pal Brian was trying to put his life back together after his divorce and suggested they choose a destination marathon so that they could run the event and holiday afterward, Craig decided he couldn't say no. After all, this was the first time in months that his friend had been excited about anything.

Craig, a 44-year-old stockbroker, had hardly run more than a few miles when he found himself completing the on-line entry form for the Venice Marathon. In the 6 months leading up to the event, he and Brian trained regularly together. Craig was surprised at how much he enjoyed the new sport and at how excited he was about the upcoming trip. The two friends planned to run the entire 26.2 miles (42 kilometers) together. Brian was by far the better runner, having run in college for Michigan State. Brian really appreciated his friend's support over the previous several months, and he wanted to celebrate their friendship by crossing the marathon finish line together.

The two guys left for Venice only days before the marathon. In hindsight, they agreed they should have allowed more time to recover from jet lag, but they had wanted to make sure they had enough time after the race to enjoy the sights of Venice. The morning of the race was sunny and warm. The two were stunned by the huge number of marathoners, as well as by all of the support along the route. Until mile 21, Craig felt great, as though the crowds and amazing scenery had helped carry him along the course. But when he had 5 miles left to complete, he felt his tank was empty. Having run most of the race, walking only through the water stations, he now told Brian to go on without him, as he needed to walk. Brian refused to leave him behind. Instead, he walked with Craig, encouraging him to keep moving and to focus on the runners in front of them. Eventually they resumed a slow jog. The pace was a little painful for Brian, as he was accustomed to running much faster, but he really wanted to cross the line with his friend, which he did. Once across, the two were overjoyed: Craig because he had run his first marathon and Brian because it was a celebration of his friendship with Craig and a positive way to deal with the loss he felt after his divorce. And it was an ideal opportunity to enjoy the sights of Venice!

easy. To keep things fresh, include some variety in the time, place, and terrain. Habits and routine are key to sticking with your marathon program, but if you aren't motivated you will begin to skip runs. For example, you may find training in your neighborhood sufficiently rewarding, but over time the experience is likely to pale. Passing the same houses, barking dogs, and coffee shops can be tedious and tiring. Avoid boredom and waning enthusiasm by planning times when you'll leave the comfort of your own community for neighboring trails and parks.

A marathon-training group or a training partner are great ways to improve motivation and stay on track. Turn to chapter 8 for more information on training groups and running partners.

Common Personality Traits of Elite Marathoners

Sport psychology research has looked at personality characteristics of high-level runners. As a whole, these individuals tend to be very goal oriented, and they maintain a consistent, steady approach toward achieving their long-term aims. They demonstrate determination and commitment to their goals, and focus more on their bodies (versus distracting themselves with external stimulus) during runs. Not surprisingly, high-level athletes use more self-talk than less experienced runners. They possess higher levels of self-awareness and use it to their advantage. Regardless of your level of experience, you can approach your running in a similar fashion.

7 You're a Runner!

YOU NOW SEE YOURSELF AS A DISTANCE RUNNER. Congratulations! If you're like many of the people who catch the running bug, you might be asking yourself how you can become a better runner. Good technique is definitely important, but there are more factors than this that can help you to improve. Strength training, stretching, and cross training form the foundation to further your running, minimize chances of injury, and increase your level of enjoyment. It may seem obvious, but if you enjoy running, you are likely to not only make it to the start line but also to become a lifelong runner.

If you use the elements outlined in this chapter, together with the guidelines set out elsewhere in this book, you will arrive at the marathon start line prepared and ready for the experience of a lifetime.

The Importance of Laying the Groundwork

The groundwork of a good running program includes two key elements: strength training and flexibility exercises. The training programs in this book use a gradual and progressive approach, but fitness varies with the individual. Age, weight, previous injuries, athletic history, and your current level of fitness are just a few of the elements to be considered when training for a marathon. A healthy 50-year-old who has spent a lifetime swimming and playing squash is starting from a different place than, for example, an overweight 45-year-old who hasn't done any exercise since high school gym class.

A regular routine of strengthening and stretching exercises alongside your training program are the building blocks for all marathoners. This is especially the case if you have been sedentary for a long period. It's like building a house: without a good foundation, the house might be able to stand upright, but chances are that it will not stand the test of time. As a marathoner with weak hip flexor muscles and tight hamstrings, you might be able to cross the finish line, but the result could be years of pain and suffering or, worse, surgery. This does not have to be the case if you implement the strength and stretching exercises outlined in this chapter.

Strength

Increasing the strength of a previously injured area will provide your joints with the support they need to keep an injury from flaring up again.

If, during the course of your training program, you become injured or experience delayed muscle soreness that lasts longer than 48 hours, it's a good idea to check with a sport medicine professional. Once you receive advice on the best approach to rehabilitating the sore or injured muscle, it's important to be patient with your recovery. As Dr. Jack Taunton of the University of British Columbia points out, "Too often, athletes return to their running program too soon after being injured. They return rested, but they have not regained the strength they need." The result is usually reinjury.

As well as helping to prevent injury and reinjury, strength training can help prevent the decrease in muscle mass that occurs with age. Increasing your strength also has some great psychological benefits: feeling strong feels good, and it makes you more confident to conquer the hills and valleys of your marathon-training runs.

Strength training

A strength-training program is an effective way to develop your muscles for running. Lower-body training strengthens your leg muscles, making your stride stronger and more powerful. Upper-body and core strength is needed for good posture and running technique. For example, if your back and abdominal muscles are weak, you will not be as erect as you could be and will have a natural tendency to lean forward, which decreases your stride and endurance. What to consider before starting a strength-training program:

1. Seek out the advice of a fitness professional. Most private gyms or community centers will provide you with contact information for someone who can help you set up a program.
2. Make sure the fitness professional who is assisting you in creating a program understands your running

Distance runners need a strong core

Core muscles include your trunk and pelvic regions. If you have weakness in your back or abdomen, distance running is going to intensify the problem. Take the time to improve the strength in the core region of your body by doing regular abdominal exercises. Yoga or Pilates classes are also great for improving the strength and flexibility of your lower-back and abdominal muscles.

goals, time demands, and any previous injuries or health care concerns.

3. Before each training session, be sure to warm up properly.

4. Include 2 or 3 training sessions per week in order to achieve optimum response.

Stretching

Runners especially need a regular stretching program for their muscles to work properly. The act of running shortens the muscles. If you regularly sit at a desk in front of a computer, it is even more important for you to stretch. Humans are not designed to sit for extended periods of time. According to Vancouver chiropractor Dr. Raffi Titizian, who works with a large number of beginning marathoners, "The combination of training for a marathon and sitting at a desk is a disaster waiting to happen. The result is short hamstrings, short hip flexors, and poor posture. The result is problems when you are erect and trying to run." Muscles that are short want to be long, but they can't be, because the brain neurologically is used to keeping them short. The result is short, tight muscles. Your muscles do not have full range of motion if they aren't flexible. Full range of motion doesn't mean being a yoga guru; it's an anatomical range of motion for your height, weight, and body type. In addition to injury prevention, increased flexibility can minimize tightness in other areas of your body, which improves running performance. The less tight and stiff you are, the better you will feel.

Stretching is essential to any running program if you

want to avoid injury. Stretching should be done after you have adequately warmed up (5 to 10 minutes of easy walking or jogging) and at the end of your cool-down session. Hip and upper-leg stretches work the pelvic and upper-leg muscle groups. Stretching the lower legs works the muscles and tendons of the lower leg and calf region. Lower-back stretches work the core area, which is the stomach and lower back.

Refer to appendix A for specific stretching exercises.

Good running form

Good running technique is usually smooth and efficient. Try not to be overly concerned with your style; you will become more comfortable, more efficient, and stronger as your running increases. Everyone has his or her individual style; even the most elite marathoners may thrash or bob, but they still manage to be effective.

Good running technique will positively affect your performance. Here are a few suggestions for optimum form:

- Remember to focus on using your arms to get the pace you want and to keep the rhythm. As you use your arms, your legs will follow.
- Let your arms swing naturally, but keep them close to your body.
- Keep your arms slightly bent at the elbows.
- Keep your hands cupped.
- Point your feet straight ahead. They should strike the ground directly underneath your hips.
- Pull your pelvis inward.
- Try to focus on running tall.

Tips on stretching

- Make sure you have properly warmed up or cooled down before starting your stretching exercises.
- Be gentle. Relax into the stretch, and avoid forcing it.
- Get into each stretch position slowly.
- Until you feel tension, gently increase the stretch.
- If it hurts, ease off, and if the pain doesn't subside, stop.
- Hold each position for 10 to 30 seconds.
- After about 10 seconds you may find the muscle relaxes, which enables you to increase the stretch.
- Develop your own sequence of stretches that become a routine part of the warm-up and cool-down portion of your training.
- Stick with light stretching as part of your warm-up, and keep the deep and longer stretching for after your run.
- Make sure you include stretches at the beginning and end of every workout.

Relax your shoulders. If the upper body and shoulders feel tight or strained, try pinching a thumb with one of your fingers. It creates a tiny pressure point and will relieve the tension in the upper body. Eventually, you'll learn to run relaxed without the pinching!

Breathing

When you exercise, you begin to breathe harder and may feel out of breath. This is natural and normal. Without giving it much conscious thought, most runners breathe in a 2:2 rhythmic ratio. They take two steps as they inhale; they take two more steps as they exhale. While running very slowly, they often breathe in a 3:3 ratio. While running very fast, they might breathe 2:1,

Maclean

Maclean, 32, is an athletic guy who had always used running as a means to stay fit for his real passions, including hockey, cycling, and windsurfing. It wasn't until he met Piper that he began to run more than once or twice a week. Piper is a competitive marathoner who runs an average of 70 miles (about 113 kilometers) per week.

Maclean started to join his new girlfriend for a few of her runs and even for the odd long run on the weekend. The only problem was that once he got up to 70 minutes, he began to experience dizziness and nausea. Because Piper didn't take in fluid or food for these runs, he felt he too should be fine. He didn't realize that it had taken her body many years of running to slowly adapt to the mileage and time on her feet. This type of running was new for Maclean. After some encouragement from Piper, he agreed to wear a waist belt in order to carry water and some sort of food replacement, such as a sport gel or bar, on their long runs. The first few times, he experienced cramping and discomfort after eating and drinking during his long run. Thinking back, he's certain he ate and drank too much, too fast. Over time, he learned to refuel and avoid cramps by taking in only small amounts of water and sport bar. He is now able to easily run for up to 2 hours, as long as he refuels throughout the long run.

or 1:1, but 2:2 is much more common. If you count breaths in and out and discover you are breathing with a different rhythm, don't worry about it. Adjusting your breathing pattern will not make you a better runner. As well, most runners and walkers naturally breathe through both mouth and nose.

Besides Running

There are many activities besides running that are fun, increase your strength and endurance, and complement your distance-running aspirations. Just about any activity that increases the flow of oxygen is considered cross training. Walking, cycling, swimming pool running, and hiking are all good ways to increase your overall fitness and add some variety to your routine. Cross training can also help your running by strengthening areas of the body that support you as you run.

How to cross train

- Give yourself a few weeks to adjust to your training program before adding cross training to the mix. Doing too much too soon could lead to injury.
- We suggest in this book's training programs you cross train on one or two of your days off from running.
- Work out once a week at your local pool.
- Consider joining a gym or your local community center.
- Pick an activity you enjoy. If you don't like getting wet, swimming or pool running might not be for you.

- If you're new to exercising, or if you've taken a long break from any form of fitness, consider walking or stretching as cross-training activities. Again, be careful not to do too much too fast. You don't want to be sidelined by an injury or burned out from too much exercise.

What cross-training activity best complements my running?

All cross-training activities will help you to increase your strength and stamina, which is valuable for running. If done correctly, running in water most closely replicates running on land.

RUNNER PROFILE

Jeanne

Jeanne had trained for four marathons, but she had never made it to the start line. Over the years she had run numerous half marathons and 10-kilometer (6.2-mile) races, but she couldn't seem to avoid injuring herself when preparing for a marathon. She had given up hope of ever making it to the marathon finish line in a healthy and safe manner. She had been tempted to run during a recent iliotibial band problem, but her friend Sacha, also a runner, strongly discouraged the idea.

Finally, after reading a book on cross training for runners, Jeanne decided she would try yoga with the hope of loosening her legs and building strength in her core. In her first class, it became clear that she was incredibly tight in key areas of her body. Without doing something to change this, the yoga instructor told her, she would continue to injure herself.

Jeanne loves running; it is not only a hobby but also a passion, and in recent years it's become a means to meditate. Jeanne may not run a marathon any time soon, but she's certain that if she sticks with her twice-weekly yoga class she has a better chance of running as she ages. And if she's lucky, one of these years she may even get to see the 26.2-mile (42-kilometer) finish line.

Here are several tips for water-running beginners:

- Imagine your own running gait. Your knee comes up in front at about a 45-degree angle, your leg extends to allow your heel to plant first, then your ankle flexes so that you can push off the ground with your toes as you drive your leg back behind you, and the opposite leg begins the cycle once again. Your lower body should follow this same pattern in the water.

- Avoid using a dog-paddle arm motion to stay afloat. Instead, concentrate on reproducing the action your arm follows when you run on land. Be sure to bring your arms straight through the water in front of you and extend them all the way back behind you, holding your hands relaxed as you do when you run.

- Start slowly. Structure your water-running program so that you gradually progress toward longer workouts. Before you dive into any of the workouts described, you should be able to comfortably handle a steady 30-minute run in the water.

- Make it as pleasant as possible. Find a pool with a large deep end or diving tank that is available at convenient times and not crowded with swimmers doing their laps or kids just playing around. That way, other swimmers won't be in your way, and you won't be in theirs. Sometimes it helps to explain to curious fellow pool users what it is you are trying to accomplish, but the best solution is to work out during quiet times of the day. Avoid lunchtime and after-work hours.

- Scout around for a pool that offers piped-in music. Music really helps pass the time as you work out.

- Find a partner. Make arrangements to meet and go for a "run" at the pool. Good conversation also helps pass the time; workouts are more fun, and there's always better motivation when someone else shares the load.

- Keep time. Use a waterproof watch to time your runs and intervals, or find a pool with a large pace clock—the kind that lap swimmers use to time their intervals.

Rachel

Rachel is a 37-year-old police officer, mother, and wife. As an elite gymnast in her younger days, she had never thought she would like running. The combination of weight training, spinning classes, and cardio workouts on the elliptical trainer at the YMCA where she worked out helped her to stay incredibly fit, but it wasn't until she met some women there that she began running.

Many of Rachel's college friends had moved away and she had found she missed having them to exercise with, so when these new friends asked her to join them for the occasional run, she didn't feel she could decline. Eventually she was joining them for several runs a week, and she entered a few local road races. She loved her new sport, and within a year she was running regularly and starting to train for a marathon. The only problem was with her lower back; after her long training runs, it would bother her for several days. She had experienced back problems in the past due to her days as a gymnast, but now it was starting to interfere with her everyday activities.

Instead of giving up on her marathon goal, Rachel researched the various cross-training options that would provide the maximum benefit for running. Everything she read suggested pool running was her best bet. In the lead-up to her marathon, she pool ran twice a week in place of shorter and medium-length runs. "I found running in the water to be a great way to build core strength, minimize my back problems, and increase my running endurance. Without pool running, I would never have made it to the marathon start line in one piece!"

Including the Family

FOR MANY ADULTS, THE ACT OF BALANCING FAMILY, HOME, and career bears all the hallmarks of a marathon: non-stop hard work. For others, training for and running 26.2 or 13.1 miles (42 or 21 kilometers) is the ultimate challenge. Without question, training for a marathon alongside the competing demands that families face requires significant planning and a lot of organizing. But it can be done. From running with a jogging stroller to finding a good training partner, this chapter provides facts on family fitness and simple strategies for busy families making it to the marathon finish line.

Marathon Women

Women's recent entry into marathoning

Much has changed for women over the past 30 years. As a result of the women's movement, the opportunities open to females in Western cultures have never been greater.

Today women work in almost all fields and professions, and it seems the woman who doesn't work outside the home is becoming the exception. The vast opportunities for women are also seen in sport, and the marathon and half marathon are great examples. Nowadays women make up over half the number of participants in most races.

Why the slow start?

Women are increasingly attracted to distance events in part because they've had a slower entry to the sport than men. Initially it was thought distance running was too taxing on the female body. As recently as the early 1970s it was commonly thought that women could not run long distances, the general assumption being that it was hazardous to women's health. In fact, numerous critiques were written by doctors warning women of the harm they would do to their bodies if they attempted to run farther than a few thousand yards. The articles suggested that women who ran long distances were likely to permanently damage their bodies. These concerns were followed by research claiming that female athletes who engaged in rigorous training schedules risked their ability to conceive children. It was not until the 1984 Olympic Games that the marathon race was sanctioned for women.

Run clinics have a big role

Vancouver International Marathon organizer Derek Hodge attributes the boom in women running half and full marathons in large part to the increasing availability of run clinics. The clinics provide a safe and simple solution for female runners, some of whom will never before have seen large groups of women running. The experience of meeting women who are faster, slower, older, or younger than you can be motivating and empowering. In contrast, women can find it discouraging if they run exclusively with men who are faster and stronger. This is not to say that there aren't superb women runners and men who make great training partners. The key is to figure out what combination works best for you.

The Marathon Clinic

Regardless of whether you're a man or woman, a marathon-training clinic can provide expert advice, guidance, and companionship on the road to achieving your marathon goal. Most running stores offer clinics, as do private fitness clubs and community centers. Clinics vary in size, cost, and general approach to marathon training, so it's important to try a few to find one that best meets your needs. Most clinics provide a free introductory session or request a nominal fee.

If you feel a little awkward or even a little intimidated at the prospect of joining a running clinic, rest assured that you're not alone. As adults we generally move in groups and within communities that we have known for years. The prospect of entering a new environment to perform an unfamiliar task is something rare and can be unnerving for even the most confident individual. Beforehand, tell yourself that at some point everyone who joins has experienced similar feelings. After a few training sessions, your uncertainty will disappear, and before you know it you will be comfortable with the other runners.

How the marathon clinic works

Prior to each training session, there is usually a short presentation by the clinic coordinator on a running-related issue such as stretching or nutrition. This is followed by a brief explanation of the upcoming training session. Afterward, participants separate into their designated pace groups. Most marathon clinics group people according to each individual's running pace; some ask that registrants list their approximate 10-kilometer running time in order to assign them to the appropriate pace group. If you are a beginner, and you don't have a clear sense of your running ability or 10-kilometer time, you may want to start in a slower group for the first few sessions. Once you complete a couple of runs with your training group, you will get a sense of which group works best for you. Runners are allowed to change groups if, for example, they improve faster than the others in the group, or if they feel the need to move to a slower group because of missed sessions.

Most people tend to push too hard right from the start of a run. Be conservative. You can always switch to a faster group, but starting too quickly and aggressively may lead to injury and frustration.

Each pace group is assigned at least one leader who will run at the front or back of the group. Clinics usually design a course that is some sort of loop, in order to allow run leaders to easily move forward or backward within the group. This way everyone still feels they are part of a group, and it minimizes the risk of participants getting lost or running at a speed that is too fast for their current fitness levels.

Marathon and Half Marathon

What to look for in a marathon-training clinic

- Make sure the clinic leaders are knowledgeable. They should understand the various elements of marathon training, such as the physical and mental demands, as well as injury-prevention and pacing strategies.
- Check that the clinic has a training program that meets your needs by inquiring as to the suggested level of fitness for their programs, and make sure you're honest with yourself regarding your current level of fitness.
- Each clinic has a different atmosphere. Some are friendlier than others, and you will learn what works best for you after trying a few.
- By visiting a clinic, you will get a sense of whether or not the coordinator is organized and punctual. If you are a busy parent or a single person with a demanding career, you may want a clinic that runs like clockwork. Some clinics are not as structured as you might prefer. This may seem a minor issue, but over the course of several months it can become incredibly frustrating.
- The location of the clinic should be a consideration. If it is conveniently located in your neighborhood or close to work, you are more likely to regularly attend the training sessions.
- If you plan to drive to the clinic, make sure there will be adequate parking. The last thing you want to do each week is spend 15 minutes searching for a parking spot before your training clinic.

Finding a Running Partner

Most marathoners would agree a good training partner is one of the most precious gifts any runner can find. Besides providing safety and security for the runner, a running cohort motivates, supports, and keeps you true to your training program. But before you ask your closest friend or spouse if he or she wants to fill this position, take some time to figure out your training needs, time limitations, and other responsibilities that will compete with your marathon schedule. Also, it's a good idea to figure out the areas in which you can be flexible. For example, you may have some leeway as to the days of the week you could join your partner, but you know the runs must occur in the morning hours before work. Once you have itemized your own needs, you can ponder which of your friends might be a good fit. At this point, consider the following questions to narrow your choice of running partner, as you want to be confident he or she can hold up one end of the partnership:

- Is she at a similar running level?
- Does he share your enthusiasm for the sport, or will you have to continually motivate him to train?
- Is he supportive of your marathon goals?
- Do you have similar schedules?
- Will it be easy and convenient to coordinate runs?
- Is she a consistent and reliable person?
- Do you enjoy spending extended periods of time with this person?

Making a plan with your running partner

Once you and your partner have agreed to try running together, it might be a good idea to start with one group run per week to establish whether the partnership will work. Make sure you organize a specific meeting place and time. Remember to be courteous and on time. It may not seem an issue to be 15 minutes late for a dinner date, but if you are regularly late in meeting your running partner, it can become a deal breaker. Waiting in the wind and rain is different from waiting inside a warm coffee shop, watching the rain beat down on the window. If you can, try to meet your partner in the foyer of a building or in a bus shelter. Some running groups have a 5- or 10-minute rule whereby they meet at a given time, and if others are not there within the set time frame they commence the run; the late party is left to his or her own devices. This is a good way of making sure that people show up on time!

Even if you have a running partner, occasionally join another friend for some extra motivation and company. He or she may accompany you on a bike, or simply drive along your route and be there for you every mile or two along the way.

Pregnancy and Running: Some Questions

Can sedentary women start running once they conceive?

The short answer is, yes! It may seem strange, but if you're a woman who was sedentary prior to becoming pregnant, now might be the time to take up a gradual

Colleen

Colleen is now a stay-at-home mom getting back into shape after having her son Kai 10 months ago. She finds that exercising on her own is what works best, giving her the flexibility to go out when she wants and to run at the speed that suits her. But this was not always the case, and as she says, her routine may change again in the future. For now, she often walks and runs with Kai in a stroller.

While Colleen was working on her doctorate in women's health, she found a great running partner in her friend Jacquie. Colleen and Jacquie would often meet several times a week. "We had similar schedules and were able to be flexible in the times we got out for our runs. Sometimes we met in the morning for a long run along the beach near my home, and other times we met at a park in Jacquie's neighborhood. As well, we were both at a similar fitness level, and most days we would run almost stride for stride. But the best part about running with Jacquie was that it meant we were able to get in a regular visit while we both maintained our busy schedules. If we didn't run together, we would have seen a lot less of each other."

and progressive walk/run program. Sport medicine physician Dr. Liz Joy of Salt Lake City, Utah, says, "It's a myth that it is dangerous for sedentary women to start exercising once they become pregnant. I encourage all of my pregnant patients to keep moving, especially the ones who are at risk of gestational diabetes." For most previously sedentary women, Dr. Joy encourages a regular walking program during the first trimester. Once the nausea—which is usually limited to the first trimester—is over, she suggests that these women take the same approach to exercise as the rest of her non-pregnant patients. Dr. Joy believes everyone, including mom and baby, can benefit from a gradual and progressive walk/run program.

Depending on how they feel, pregnant women can begin a gradual walk/jog program, perhaps working up to a 5- or 10-kilometer (3- or 6-mile) distance, but this is definitely not the time to embark on a half- or full-marathon journey.

Is distance running safe for pregnant women?

We don't have to look very far to see pregnant women exercising. Whether it's at our local yoga studio, swimming pool, or jogging track at our community center, women are choosing to stay active during pregnancy. However, marathoning women need to look for a balance between staying healthy while pregnant and not pushing themselves too hard. Dr. Karen Nordahl, physician and co-author of the pre-natal fitness book *Fit to Deliver*, says, "A woman can run as long as she feels comfortable and has no pregnancy or orthopedic complications." It has been found that women who were regular runners before becoming pregnant often find they can run long into their pregnancies.

Can I continue to train for a marathon during my pregnancy?

Dr. Joy says pregnancy is not the time to improve your fitness level for a future marathon. Instead, she encourages women to focus on staying healthy and active. Being active means different things to different women. For example, a woman who was sedentary prior to pregnancy would likely find a gradual walk/run program to be the ideal challenge. For elite marathoners, running at a moderate pace several times a week is likely achievable. Although there are no specific guidelines for how much or how little running is safe for pregnant women, Dr. Nordahl suggests that if you ran regularly before becoming pregnant, and you don't have any complications, you could continue running until 8 to 10 weeks before your delivery date. Be certain to monitor your exertion level, and only run at a moderate pace. Also advise your health care provider of your exercise routine. If you are fit and have done a significant amount of distance running prior to pregnancy, you still should ask your doctor for the green light to continue training. As you know, each pregnancy is unique, so it's important to be responsible and plan according to the guidelines provided by a health care professional.

When can new mothers begin training for a marathon?

If you're wanting to continue or start a half- or full-marathon program post-pregnancy, it's essential that you take a gradual and progressive approach. Your body has been through a lot. You need to be well rested and recovered from your pregnancy before starting an aggressive training regime. If you start back too soon or take an overly aggressive approach, it increases the likelihood of injury and extreme fatigue. Because of this, health care providers recommend that you check in with them for specific guidelines that will work for you. However, as a general rule, it's good to wait at least two weeks after a vaginal birth and 6 to 8 weeks after a cesarean section before returning to a regular running schedule. As a means of easing your body back into running, you may want to start with some fast walking, then progress to faster walking, and gradually you will be jogging and running as your body adjusts and is ready for it.

Do lactating marathoners need to take any special precautions?

Hydration and finding a good sport bra are essential for lactating runners. During pregnancy and beyond, it is especially important for women to remain well hydrated, especially if they're breast feeding. Take along a water bottle, or include a water stop on all of your runs, even the shorter ones.

Given that your breasts will have increased in size and tenderness (if you're breast feeding), a good sport bra is essential. But finding one that provides comfort and function and minimizes movement can be difficult. Some women have found that because of extra sensitivity and density of the breast, they prefer a bra that eliminates all or most of the movement in the breast area. Most bra and sportswear companies provide a good selection of exercise bras that meet the needs of all women, regardless of shape and size. Ask your local running store for suggestions on good running bras. If they don't have one that meets your needs, it's likely they will be able to suggest a brand and store that does.

Marathoning Families

There's little doubt that taking on the challenge of training for and completing a half or full marathon will affect almost every aspect of your life. Your diet, your sleep patterns, your relationships, and your work will almost certainly be realigned and reshaped along the way. Viewed by some as a crime of selfishness, marathon training doesn't have to be a felony if you are committed to making it work for you and your family. The following section provides tips, suggestions, and tools for making the marathon experience a positive one for you and your loved ones.

Why the marathon?

It's important to share with your family some of your reasons for wanting to take on such a colossal endeavor as the marathon. It is especially important if you weren't a regular runner in the past. Don't expect your spouse and others to be immediately supportive. Sometimes it takes time for others to fully understand our marathon aspirations.

Make sure it's the right time

Ask yourself if it is the best time for you to pursue your marathon goal. If your wife is about to have a baby, or you're tutoring your daughter for 3 hours every night to prepare her for her SATS, it may not be the best time to spend several extra hours a week away from your home and family. Waiting for the right time for those close to you increases the likelihood of gaining your family's support and, in turn, meeting your marathon goal. You want to do everything you can to enjoy the experience and not view it as simply another source of stress.

Getting organized

Organization is key when it comes to marathon training. Running four times a week takes a significant amount of time. In order to stick to your training program, you need to organize all of the important areas of your life. Take the time to sit down with your spouse and discuss any upcoming events such as birthdays and weddings, as well as potential concerns. Using a calendar and your training program, begin making a household plan that looks after the needs of your home and family and still allows you to fulfill the demands of your marathon program. Here are some things to consider when making your plan:

- Establish the days and times when you can fit in each of your week's runs. Pencil these runs into a family calendar, and post it in a central location so that everyone can support mom and/or dad's next training run.
- Decide who is responsible for each of the household

chores, such as laundry, cleaning, grocery shopping, paying bills, carpooling, and child care. Once you've delegated each task, decide when it will be done. This may sound overly organized, but creating a detailed plan at the onset of one's training program will reduce stress, confusion, and conflict during the months of marathon preparation.

- Plan your weekly menu and grocery list. This is not the time to be making extravagant dinners, but that doesn't mean meals cannot be healthy and tasty.
- Be sure to build in some extra rest after each long run. Your long runs will take a lot out of you. You may want to schedule an afternoon nap or some

Steven

Steven is a 42-year-old business lawyer and a single father who runs four times a week. A rugby player in college, he ran to stay fit. It wasn't until he was practicing law that he began to run for pleasure and as a means of de-stressing. After meeting his wife and having two children, Steven began running with the baby jogger. "Using the stroller, having to plan the timing of runs, and having the opportunity to get the babies out of the house and quiet for a few hours actually helped me get some focus. It definitely was not a detriment."

Over the years, Steven has run seven marathons, and much of his training was done with the jogging stroller. Today, he runs on his own after work and on weekends when he has the kids. With a little cajoling, the children often agree to accompany him on their bikes. "Having the kids cycle alongside isn't always easy; they often want to stop, and the pace can be a problem. But if we visit new parks and neighborhoods it seems they have more fun, are more focused on riding, and less concerned about the upcoming hill. Regardless, training with my kids is a great motivator and a wonderful way to spend and afternoon." These days, Steven is training for the Paris Marathon. His kids won't travel to France, but they will definitely be supporting him during some of his long training runs.

easy chores. You don't want to be cutting the grass or teaching your daughter how to ride a bike after your 3-hour run. Fatigue not only limits energy—it can also decrease your patience.

- Encourage family members to join you for the odd run. If they aren't runners, suggest they roller-blade or bike alongside you. Or they can meet you at the end of a long run; go out for ice cream as a celebration. By including family and friends in your training, you will make them feel part of the team.

- If you have a running partner or a running group, plan a post-run dinner or breakfast that involves your family. It's good to be excited about new friends and shared goals, but your family also wants to be part of the excitement. Sharing the ups and downs of your training with loved ones helps you to remain connected throughout the marathon experience.

Children in the Training Equation

Children learn about exercise from their parents, and pediatrician Dr. Trent Smith encourages parents to include children in their training equation. Kids are like sponges. By running with a jogging stroller, having your daughter join you on a bike, or meeting your teenage son for a lemonade after a long run, you're modeling good behavior for your child. Studies show that families who play together and make exercise a regular part of their lives are more likely to have children who view exercise as an everyday activity.

Marathon training with a jogging stroller

The jogging stroller can be an essential item for marathoning moms and dads, but pushing a jogging stroller for an hour-long run is more difficult than it looks. Even for the extremely fit, it takes time to build the strength, comfort, and coordination required to run with a stroller. You might want to start with a gradual walk/run and gradually build up your comfort level before attempting a short or medium-length run.

Once you're comfortable running with a jogging stroller, it's a great way to have time with your baby and get out for your midweek runs. But having your baby with you for your long runs might be too much for both of you. Dr. Liz Joy recommends that parents trust their instincts when it comes to the acceptable amount of time a baby can sit comfortably in the jogging stroller. Some parents find that taking a rest break halfway through a run is a great way to keep both parent and child happy. Consider stopping at a park and allowing your baby to enjoy the new surroundings while you refuel and catch your breath.

Be realistic about your children. Having your child with you on a bike or in a jogger can be very rewarding, but for a marathon and half-marathon program it is unlikely they will be great companions for the longer runs. Make sure you can count on some child care during that time.

Making your child's health a priority

If your children are beyond the jogging stroller phase, there are a lot of great ways for them to share your marathon experience. If your child expresses an interest in joining you on a run, encourage him or her to accompany you on a bike. After watching you run, your child may become interested in joining you on foot. If this is the case, make sure the focus is on having fun. Try

Paige

Paige is a 13-year-old who has always preferred reading and drawing to any kind of sport. She's a shy girl and usually spends most of her free time working on her next art creation; for the past couple of years, she has had a huge fascination with unicorns and has won several prizes in youth drawing contests across the U.S. It's not that she dislikes exercise—in fact, she often goes for evening walks with her mother. But at school Paige feels intimidated by team sports. She doesn't know many of the other kids, and when she's in gym class she's usually sitting on the sidelines or is one of the last to be picked for teams.

Now that Paige is becoming a teenager and interested in boys, she's increasingly aware of her growing body. She is determined to lose the extra weight she seems to have gained in the past year. Her increasing waistline can, at least in part, be attributed to hormones and the normal changes most adolescents face, but she cannot ignore her poor diet and minimal exercise. At a recent checkup, Paige asked her family physician to suggest a good diet that would promote weight loss. She was surprised to hear that diet alone would not help her lose pounds, nor maintain a healthy weight. The doctor also told her that if she were to continue down her current path of minimal exercise and excessive fast food, she would likely become obese before the age of 20. This really scared Paige and made her even more resolved to lose the extra weight. She decided to take her doctor's advice to try a walk/run program.

Paige is now 3 months into that program and very pleased with her commitment to exercise. She hasn't lost quite as much weight as she would like, but it's slowly coming off and staying off. She recently completed her first 5-kilometer race and is now training for a 10-kilometer event. She feels healthier and happier with her decreased cravings for fast food, and she has made friends who join her for most of her walk/run sessions. What started out as a weight-loss program has turned into a life-altering experience. Paige still enjoys her artwork, but she doesn't miss her sedentary lifestyle.

exploring your local park, and incorporate a walk/run game. Dr. Smith says, "By making exercise play-driven, kids are more likely to be inspired to exercise regularly. If children see running as something that is only hard work, it is unlikely that they will want to make it a regular habit that will last into their teen and adult years."

Kids who want to train for a half or full marathon

As your children watch you train for your marathon, there is a chance they will catch the running bug. You don't want to quash their enthusiasm and passion for running, but sport physicians and pediatricians agree that training for and completing a marathon is too demanding for anyone under 18 years of age. When helping your pre-adolescent child with his or her running goals, it's best to use common sense. The Canadian Pediatrics Association says there are no clear guidelines for this group of runners. Dr. Smith suggests that running a 10-kilometer race might be too much for a child, but a grade 5 or 6 student who has run a couple of 5-kilometer races probably could, with some training, run a 10-kilometer race.

Your keen, active child can be safely encouraged to accompany you on the two shorter workout days in our program, under which you will both be gradually progressing to a 10-, 12-, and 20-minute jog over a 20-week period.

Helping your sedentary child to safely become more active

Whether your child is 10 or 15 years of age, there is little scientific literature on which to base recommendations for adolescent running programs. To minimize the risk of injury and future concerns, strength and conditioning experts recommend sequential training programs for adolescents. If it's running that interests your child, start him or her with a gradual walk/run program. Using blocks of 3 to 4 weeks, your child can gradually increase the running time. Before that happens, it's a good idea to evaluate how he or she is responding to the program. You can do this by timing him or her over a measured distance. If running times are increasing rather than decreasing, the young runner is likely fatigued and possibly needs an extra rest day to recover. In the beginning, running times should stay the same or gradually decrease. Remember, every person progresses at distinct rates. It's also a good idea to monitor children for potential signs of injury by asking them a series of questions every week or so. The questions should include the following:

- How do you feel?
- Are you tired?
- How do your legs feel?
- How do your feet feel?
- How does your back feel?

If they are experiencing some pain, ask them to localize it. These questions might seem straightforward to most adults, but you have to remember that structured exercising—and the discomfort that can be associated with such exercise—is completely new for your child. Articulating how he or she is feeling can be difficult, which is why you need to probe for feedback on training progress. If the youngster is experiencing pain, set up a rest day or two. If the soreness doesn't dissipate within a couple of days, make an appointment for the young runner to see your sport medicine physician.

Including the Household

Congratulations, you've taken the first step and made a personal commitment to train for the half or full marathon. Now comes the task of figuring out the best times to train, given the demands of the household. Within a typical busy family, your running will require the support of that helpful spouse, partner, or close friend, or it may require spending a little money on child care. The key is to develop a pattern for your workouts. Write down your options in your daytimer, in a diary, or on a wall calendar. Organize child care, and stick to it. Your workouts must be structured, or they will not happen!

Overcome your child care anxieties by searching out a local gym or community center where child care is provided for a reasonable price. It takes time and patience to organize what your pre-schooler needs at day care. Accept that there will be a few "unhappy" sessions before your child gets used to the new environment.

Child care at your local gym won't work as your longer workouts become too long, but it's a terrific option for your two shorter sessions. If your children don't do well in child care or if cost is an issue, you may need to search out a partner, friend, or neighbor with whom you can switch child care responsibilities. You can watch their child or do their shopping in return for their watching your children while you run.

Tips for organizing work, kids, and distance running

- Being a parent is the most important job of all, and taking the time to work out can be challenging. You might want to consider using your lunch hour to fit in your weekly runs. If you need a little extra time, perhaps speak with your boss and organize yourself so that you can eat a bag lunch at your desk.

- Perhaps you can utilize your workout as your mode of transportation, alternating traveling by foot to work one day, and home from work on another. You'll have to organize your clean, dry clothing and necessary toiletries at your workplace, but it's possible. And chances are you'll feel great about using your legs instead of your car.

- Start your weekend long run early so that you can still enjoy the bulk of the day with family.

- If your children are older, be sure to have a discussion with them about the demands of your program, what you'll need from them, and what it will mean in terms of the household. Give them the opportunity to make suggestions as to how they can help.

- Have your teen make a commitment to take care of a younger sibling once a week during your workout.

- Have your older children take turns preparing a simple dinner for the family on the nights that you run. It's a good time for them to learn how to be creative in the kitchen, anyway! It's our job as parents to teach our children some culinary skills.

- Create a family chore schedule together, so that the duties are shared. Perhaps the vacuuming and dusting get done while you're doing your workout once a week.

- If your teen can drive, have him or her take other siblings to their extracurricular activities. If not, don't be afraid to ask neighbors and friends to help. Shared carpooling is the answer. Again, take the time to make a routine for yourself so that everybody can adjust to the changes and your commitment.

- The family that works together and shares together stays together and learns to appreciate one another. Your marathon journey can strengthen your family as easily as it can cause resentment.

Family meal planning

- Keeping enough food in the house and consistently planning healthy meals is always a challenge. Now is not the time to plan gourmet meals. Prepare a large batch of pasta sauce or soup so that leftovers can be easily warmed in the microwave.

- Now is the time to look at the staple foods in your local supermarket with new eyes. If you can't manage the shopping, have your partner support you by doing the big-bulk shop once every couple of weeks so that you can get your long workout in and to ensure there is enough food for the week.

- Fresh produce, vegetables, pastas, and breads are simple and healthy options for you and your family. It takes only minutes to make spaghetti with a simple tomato sauce. Try to avoid packaged fast-food items that are packed with fat and preservatives.

- Grabbing a piece of fruit on the go is a much better choice than a handful of cookies. To feel your best, you must commit to making healthy food choices.

Running with the Family Dog

Reliable, committed, and quiet. For many runners, the family dog is the best training partner they could find. But, like humans, not all dogs are created equal. As you can imagine, some breeds are better suited for running than others.

Finding a good running dog

Generally, a good running dog has a medium build, weighs between 50 and 70 pounds (about 22 to

32 kilograms) and has medium-short hair. Breeds such as retired greyhounds, Labradors and other retrievers, setters, spaniels, and working dogs such as Border collies and huskies make good running dogs. As well, some crossbreeds can make great running companions. If you live in a warm climate, it may be important to know that black-coated dogs do not fare well in a hot and humid climate.

Kathy

Kathy is a 55-year-old family physician and mother of four beautiful daughters. This year her youngest daughter, Em, will graduate from high school and head off to university. Kathy and her husband, Pete, will be on their own for the first time since the early days of their marriage.

Kathy had run regularly a couple of times a week but always preferred swimming and windsurfing. She would occasionally run with one of her daughters, but for company she usually relied on her faithful pooch, Baily, a golden retriever. Kathy was always pleased to see her daughters joining their dad on runs. Initially, it was just around the block; later, as the girls grew and became crazy about soccer and cross-country running, they would run farther. Finally, as university and high school athletes, the four girls, now faster and fitter than their father, would drag him out for part of their long runs while home on vacation.

It always looked as if they were having so much fun, and many inside jokes were lost on mom. Secretly, Kathy always wanted to join in, but she told herself this was something the kids did with their dad. After all, it was Pete who was the great runner.

Kathy had done one local 10-kilometer race but didn't find it very enjoyable. So when she turned 55 and announced to her daughters that she was training for a half marathon, they were more than a little surprised. Kathy had decided it would be her year to do some of the things she had put off while the kids were growing. The two items at the top of her list were hiking the challenging West Coast Trail on Vancouver Island in British Columbia and running a half marathon with her daughters Laura and Care.

How to train your dog to run with you

Depending on the size of your dog, you should wait between 6 months and 1 year before introducing it to running. If you have a larger-breed dog you should wait at least a year before including it in our running program. According to veterinarian Dr. Nicky Parkinson, of Victoria, B.C., "The reason for the discrepancy is that larger-breed dogs mature over a longer period of time. For example, a small-breed dog will often come into heat before a larger-breed dog at the same age."

At first her family thought Kathy's goals were just part of a midlife crisis that would pass with time. She thought otherwise. She went on-line and found a half-marathon training schedule that would give her guidance and a newfound confidence to push her farther than she had thought possible. She did most of her training alone but shared her aches and pains with her daughters over the phone. She was surprised when the girls began asking her about her training. She was beginning to feel like a real runner.

On the day of her half marathon, Kathy was nervous and uncertain she would be able to complete the distance. But Laura, an elite runner, gave her comfort by saying that she and Care would walk with her when needed and go at a pace that worked. This was all Kathy needed to hear. The first 10 kilometers felt great, but then Kathy took in too much water and began to get a cramp. After walking for a few minutes, she was ready to resume running. With the exception of also walking up a small hill, she ran the entire half-marathon course and was thrilled to cross the finish line with two of her daughters.

Kathy was tired after the race, but more than anything she soaked in the euphoria of achieving her distance-running goal with her daughters alongside and cheering her on for the entire 13.1 miles. Her running goal may have been part of a midlife crisis, but it was also a way for Kathy to connect with her daughters and experience some of the excitement and fun she had watched for so many years.

Once your dog is old enough to run, most veterinarians suggest a gradual introduction to running with you. For the first few weeks, have your dog run no more than 3 miles at a time, then gradually build up the running time over the course of several months.

Warning signs that your dog has done too much

Be aware of increased saliva, vomiting, irregular breathing, or an uneven gait. If you notice these signs, stop your dog and take a break. If the symptoms persist, take your pet to the vet to be checked out.

Lameness in dogs that run

If you ignore the warning signs that your dog is overdoing it, you can risk injuring your pup. Dr. Parkinson says, "Many owners don't always appreciate their animal is lame until it is at an acute level. Keep in mind, dogs will run even when they are lame. Watch for a slowing of the pace over time during a run, or an inability to complete a route the dog is normally able to do with ease. As well, some dogs will change their eating habits when they are in pain; their appetite may decrease, or they might become choosier about the food they will eat. If you notice any of these signs, take the dog to your veterinarian and have a checkup.

Pitfalls and Potential Problems

RESTED AND READY TO RUN... WHEN IT COMES TO PREPAR-
ing for a half or full marathon, there is a fine balance between training enough and training too much. One of the most difficult
aspects of marathon training is to make it to the start line rested and
injury free. Training for a distance event is demanding for even the
fittest folk.

The programs in this book are designed to minimize your
chances of suffering a running-related injury while training for your
half or full marathon. You can, however, still be sidelined as a result
of an illness, overzealous training, or your own biomechanical weak-
nesses. In order to remain healthy, it is important to understand
and incorporate some basic injury-prevention strategies into your
training. As you make your way through your program, you will
likely notice an increasing awareness of your body. With some simple guidelines, you will be able to detect the difference between a
sore muscle and a more serious pain that has potential for injury.

- Go at your own pace. If you're in a marathon clinic, don't be pressured into going too fast just to keep up with the group. Take the first couple of weeks to experiment with different pace groups. And don't be concerned about dropping back to a slower group if you have an off day or if you just cannot keep up.

- Use the talk test as a way to judge your own pace. You want to find a pace that allows you to comfortably hold a conversation with your training partner. If you cannot speak four or five consecutive sentences without feeling winded, you're going too fast and need to slow down.

- Start slowly. Trust and follow your marathon-training schedule—you will be properly guided and avoid doing too much, too soon. Remember that it takes time to learn to run, and it takes time for your body to adapt to the stresses you place on it.

Avoid Inconsistent Training

A slow, gradual, and deliberate approach is by far the safest way to train for a marathon. But it's easy to get overzealous. It's especially common for beginners to take the approach that more training is better. For first-timers, more running usually translates to more chances of injury. This is why we suggest you take a graduated approach to training and avoid dramatic increases in the amount of running you do from one week to the next.

If you ask, any sport medicine physician will tell you that the leading cause of injuries for new exercisers is running too far, or too fast, before they're ready. Your focus should be on making it to the start line healthy and ready to run. Avoid getting caught up over the total miles you run midweek or the speed at which you finish each of your sessions. Your long run is the only session for which we recommend measuring and keeping track of your distance. For more information on your long run, return to chapter 3. Beginners often have difficulty understanding the time and patience required to become a marathoner. Elite runners, for example, will train for and race shorter-distance races like 5- and 10-kilometer (3- and 6-mile) events before even contemplating the half- or full-marathon distances.

To be successful in the marathon, you need to do your homework. This means following the suggested three sessions per week. If the first few weeks of your program seem too easy, rest assured the workload does increase and will become too difficult if you haven't properly completed the sessions in the weeks before.

Try to make the appointment with yourself to do your workouts, stick to it, and resist the temptation to jump ahead in the schedule. Inconsistency can also be problematic. Skipping a workout and then adding an extra session to the following week's training schedule in an effort to make up for the lost workout is dangerous. It is also not advisable to cram your three weekly sessions into consecutive days. Instead, plan ahead, and space your runs evenly throughout the week.

Don't be concerned if you miss the odd session throughout your training program. Life is busy, and there are many competing demands for our time. If you miss a session one week, try not to worry; tell yourself you will be back on track next week. Again, remember to avoid running on consecutive days. The risks of injury far outweigh the benefits of getting in that extra run.

Common Reasons for Injuries

Running with pain

If something hurts, don't try to "run through it." Always listen to your body. Pain is a warning sign that should not be ignored. In the beginning, there will always be a few aches and pains that come with starting any new activity. However, they should dissipate within 24 to 48 hours. If they don't, or if the pain intensifies, seek professional assistance. Early identification and treatment of an injury will result in minimal interruptions to your training schedule. It's important to listen to your body and distinguish between an ache and a pain. An ache is a low-level discomfort associated with exercising; a pain is a sharp discomfort that can be localized. This is not to say that you should ignore the aches that accompany running.

Not sticking with your schedule

The most common running injury is overuse, or chronic injury that can result from overtraining. Dr. Jim Macintyre, a sport physician in Salt Lake City, says many overuse injuries result either from incomplete rehabilitation of an old injury or from individual anatomical variations that lead to injury when put under stress. The results are the same: when there's a weak link in the kinetic (moving) chain—some part that's not moving properly as the result of an injury—the other joints and muscle tendon units will compensate, leading to overload of another site as the runner tries to keep going. This usually leads to a different, new injury. For Dr. Macintyre, the red flags go up when runners go to him suffering from a cycle of injuries to one side of their body.

Choosing a poor training surface

Injuries for runners are often the result of impact, overuse, or pushing yourself too hard. A contributing factor is training on hard surfaces, which increases the level of impact on your body. The majority of runners log the most miles on asphalt. This is not the softest surface, but it is easier on your joints than concrete. Try to run or walk on the most level part of the road or pathway. Cambered roads will lead to imbalance and possibly injury. Try to log some of your miles on softer terrain such as grass or dirt trails, but remember, when you're doing your off-road runs, you need to look out for things like hard-to-see bumps, holes, sprinklers, and tree roots.

Returning to running too soon following an injury

Many runners, especially those with a specific goal such as a marathon in their sights, frequently endanger their immediate or future health by returning to action too soon after injury. Not allowing yourself to complete your rehabilitation program can potentially lead to more injuries. New injuries, notes Dr. Macintyre, can also be caused by old injuries that haven't healed properly. An ankle sprain, for example, might result in a loss of motion at the subtalar joint of the foot, which controls pronation and supination. Dr. Macintyre says he's looked at thousands of people with one pronated foot and one supinated foot, and at first he thought it odd that these people were born like that. "But the truth is, they weren't born like that. Somewhere along the way, something happened to the ankle that changed the range of motion or flexibility. The alignment was thrown out of balance, and the rest of the links in the chain started to compensate. Before the person started running, they may never have noticed this."

Sadly, some runners get into a cycle of injuries and eventually throw in the towel. "I used to run," you'll hear them say, "but my [fill in the blank] couldn't take it." Maybe it couldn't, but more than likely these runners didn't have a proper diagnosis of the problem or follow the right course of treatment.

If you do sustain an injury, and if you don't see fairly

rapid improvement from some initial self-treatment, get help from a professional who understands sport injuries. Sport medicine is not a strict discipline in the way cardiology or neurology are, but an increasing number of physicians focus on sport-related injuries. Other practitioners who may focus on such injuries include podiatrists, chiropractors, physiotherapists, athletic therapists, athletic trainers, and massage therapists. You will benefit most from someone who will examine the entire chain of your moving parts—someone who can assess the body of motion and not just look at localized pain.

Most Common Injuries

Dr. Jack Taunton, a sport medicine physician at the University of British Columbia's Allan McGavin Sport Medicine Centre, says, "It is normal for beginning marathoners to experience some degree of muscle soreness." Use the 2-day rule: if you're still feeling some degree of soreness 2 days after a training session, take an extra rest day, or do a cross-training activity like swimming or some easy cycling that is non–weight bearing.

Information to prevent injuries

By following the programs in this book—giving sufficient time to warming up and cooling down, watching where you are going, and investing in proper footwear, not to mention feeding your body properly and keeping it hydrated—you are going a long way toward preventing injury. Nevertheless, injuries occur, so it's best to be prepared. Dr. Taunton says beginning runners, not

Table 11

Area	Injury	Description	Cause	Treatment
Knee	**Iliotibial band syndrome** (the iliotibial band is a strip of connective tissue running from the hip and down the outside of the leg to just below the knee)	Pain along the outside of the knee, particularly when weight bearing on a slightly bent leg. The connective tissue becomes irritated as it rubs back and forth across the bone at the outside of the knee.	Poor shoes, hard running surfaces, repeated bending and straightening of the knee, biomechanical weakness, or inability to absorb shock.	Short-term: RICE (see next page). Long-term: regular warm-up and stretching, softer shoes to absorb the shock, avoidance of hard running surfaces and cambered routes.
Knee	**Patello-femoral syndrome** (commonly known as runner's knee)	Pain at the inner and outer part of the kneecap.	Overuse, excessive ankle pronation (inward rotation of foot), muscular imbalance around the kneecap itself.	Short-term: RICE (see next page). Long-term: correct footwear, muscle flexibility and strength, possibly orthotics.
Shin	**Tibial stress syndrome** (commonly referred to as shin splints)	Irritation along the inside front edge of the tibia (big bone in the lower leg), aching, throbbing, and/or tenderness along the inside of the shin. Particularly noticeable at the beginning of the workout; tends to subside once you've warmed up. Gets worse with time.	Minute tears in the muscles where they attach to the shin, caused by excessive pronation, too much shock to the lower extremity, inadequate flexibility, or an old injury.	Short-term: RICE (see next page); reduce your running until you are pain free. Long-term: orthotics and stretching and strengthening of the muscles in the lower leg.
Feet	**Plantar fasciitis** (the plantar fascia is a band of connective tissue running from heel to toes on the sole of the foot)	A pain in the foot, often worse in the morning. Often feels like a bruised heel; direct pressure hurts.	Overuse injury brought on by a sudden increase in frequency or intensity of training; excessive pronation, inflexible, weak foot musculature.	Short-term: RICE (see next page). Long-term: softer footwear, possibly orthotics. Train on softer surfaces; strengthening and stretching helps.
Ankle	**Achilles tendonitis**	Burning sensation and dull or sharp pain along the back of the calf, especially on the tendon. Some redness or sensation of heat may be present along the tendon itself.	Small tears that develop as a result of overuse; inflammation and resulting formation of scar tissue (adhesions) prevent the tendon from functioning optimally.	Short-term: RICE (see next page). Long-term: a more stable shoe that controls foot motion, orthotics, and increased flexibility and strength in the feet, calves, and shins.

surprisingly, experience injuries primarily in the lower parts of the body: hips, knees, shins, ankles, and feet.

RICE

RICE stands for Rest, Ice, Compression, and Elevation. It is a common and effective procedure that is often used alongside anti-inflammatory medications such as ibuprofen (Advil or Motrin). Anti-inflammatories are used to reduce swelling but should not be used to mask pain in order to train through injuries.

Rest is essential to keep an injury from getting worse. This doesn't mean you should stop all activity. In fact, complete immobility is rarely recommended. Stimulating blood flow to the injured soft tissue is necessary for healing. Speak with your sport medicine practitioner for recommendations on how best to strengthen the muscles around the injured area. Also ask about ways to increase flexibility and enhance circulation in and around the area.

Ice is a great way to decrease swelling, minimize pain from an injury, and speed recovery time. Apply ice as quickly as possible, and do so for approximately 20 minutes at a time. Allow for at least an hour between treatments. Make sure you place a thin layer of wet cloth (for example, a tensor bandage) between the bag of ice and your skin. It is best to use crushed ice, but when it is not available, gel cold packs or even a frozen bag of peas can be used. Take care when using any chemical-style packs.

Compression using an elastic wrap such as a tensor bandage can prevent swelling, reduce pain, and minimize bruising. Compression needs to be firm but not too tight. The process is extremely effective when combined with ice and elevation. A compression bandage should not be left on for longer than 3 hours and never left on overnight.

Elevation refers to elevating the injured area above the heart, which minimizes pooling of the blood and therefore reduces the swelling of the injured area.

Orthotics

What are orthotics?

A Vancouver podiatrist, Dr. Joseph Stern, describes custom orthotics as a functional and correctional device to help in prevention and treatment of injuries, biomechanical abnormalities, and anatomical misalignment. The realignment of the muscles, tendons, and joints allows the foot to be more efficient. If the bones are not in proper alignment, there can be stress on the tendons and joints that, if left untreated, can lead to problems in the feet, back, or hips. To minimize, stop, or even reverse these problems, the foot needs to be placed in a neutral position. The neutral position is attained with the use of custom orthotics, which are placed by hand into the footbed of your shoe and can be easily removed and used in other shoes.

What is the difference between orthotics bought in a running store and ones that are custom-made?

Store-bought orthoics are known as over-the-counter arch supports. These are accommodative devices that provide some cushioning and minimal control. They

How to prevent injuries

- Forget fashion. Find shoes that fit you and meet your biomechanical needs.
- Don't jump ahead in your training schedule. A gradual and progressive approach is best when it comes to distance running.
- Listen to what your body is telling you. If it hurts, back off. If the pain persists for more than 48 hours, be sure to see a sport medicine practitioner.
- Take a day off if you're feeling under the weather, and rest until you're feeling back to normal.

are not specific to one's foot, but they are a starting point to establish whether an insert is helpful. In creating a custom orthotic, a podiatrist will examine the lower extremities (hips and knees), provide a gait analysis, and complete a biomechanical analysis of the feet. This examination includes reviewing a foot's range of motion, muscle strength, and positioning.

Will it take time to get used to orthotics?

Orthotics require a period of adjustment. Start by wearing them on an easy 20- or 30-minute walk. Once you're comfortable walking, you can begin wearing them for 10 or 15 minutes during an easy run. Gradually increase your running time by 5 or 10 minutes. Breaking in orthotics can cause various types of pain in the feet, ankles, knees, legs, hips, or back. If this happens, see your podiatrist for a possible modification of your orthotic.

Should I take my orthotics with me when I buy running shoes?

Before you purchase new runners, try them on with your orthotics. Make sure the orthotics don't slip around in the runners; they should fit snuggly into the shoe.

How long do custom-made orthotics last?

Most orthotics will last 5 to 6 years, but the additional padding can be changed when needed.

The Injury-Awareness Scale

Imagine a scale between 1 and 10; "1" represents very little awareness of pain, and "10" represents an extremely high awareness of pain. Your injury-awareness level needs to be down to 2 or 3 before it's safe for you to return to activity, and it should not increase to a higher rating as a result of returning to activity. Ideally, your level of pain awareness should decrease to 1 or 2. If your awareness increases, return to cross training until it settles down. Be sure to monitor yourself honestly and carefully, and talk to your sport medicine physician for guidance in making your decision to take time off.

When it comes to injuries, it's very important for you to be honest with yourself. If you've returned to training and your injury/pain awareness starts to increase again, this is a serious indication that your body needs more recovery time. Only you can truly judge what you feel, and it's much better to take an extra week or two to rest than to risk doing serious damage to yourself. Too many people resume activity before complete recovery from injury. The result is often further time off or, worse yet, a more serious injury. If this happens to you, discuss your recovery plan with your sport medicine practitioner in order to establish the flaw in your previous process.

Coping with the Psychological Effects of an Injury

Vancouver sport psychologist Dr. David Cox says that if you're well into your marathon-training program and starting to enjoy the benefits of an active lifestyle, chances are you will have to overcome a sometimes-lengthy adjustment period after an injury. "The adjustment period is characterized by five stages: denial and isolation, anger, bargaining, depression, and acceptance." An injury that stops or slows your marathon training can cause harm to your emotional health and well-being. Here are a few suggestions for minimizing the emotional lows:

1. Seek professional advice to create a rehabilitation plan that meets your needs.

2. Make a detailed plan to stay active while injured.

3. Consider various cross-training activities that are of interest to you.

4. If you normally run after work, make sure you fill that time with one of your cross-training activities.

5. Look at this time as an opportunity to try a new activity and a chance to strengthen areas that complement your running. For example, weight training or yoga will help build your core muscles, which are essential to good posture and running technique.

6. Continue to meet up with your running partners. If you usually go for breakfast after your weekend long run, plan to cross train and then meet them afterward. This way, you won't feel grumpy for having missed out on a run, and you can share with them aspects of your cross-training activity while catching up on what's new with their marathon training.

7. Remember, most people experience an injury from time to time. When you return from your injury, you will be rested, wiser, and ready to run!

The Uncomfortable Aspects of Running

Blisters

Blisters may seem a minor issue in comparison with an injury, but any runner will tell you that a blister, especially one left untreated, can really slow you down. Once a blister develops, it doesn't take long before you find yourself cutting short a workout. If left untreated, a blister can easily become infected, forcing you to take several days off training. The good news is that they're easy to care for and avoid. Proper running shoes, socks, inserts, and petroleum jelly such as Vaseline all minimize the formation of blisters. Before a long run, apply a thick coat of Vaseline over your entire foot. This will reduce friction and prevent hot spots. Another suggestion is to reduce calluses with a pedicure file so that you can get at and treat new blisters that develop.

Tips for handling blisters

- Sock seams often blister feet. If this is the case for you, try wearing your socks with the seam facing out.

- Visit your local drugstore and check in the first-aid section for "second skin" products. They are literally a synthetic "skin," and when placed over your blister, coupled with a good adhesive strip, will bind and protect the area until the new skin is formed.

- Apply an antibiotic ointment to the blister, add a good adhesive plaster, and finally, stick a strong strip of duct tape directly over the tender area. It won't breathe and needs to be removed after your run, but it offers the best on-the-spot protection.

Ingrown nails

Ingrown toenails can be nasty. Square off the edges of your toenails, get rid of any rough edges with a nail file, and file down the centers of your nails so that they are quite thin. This takes the pressure off the nasty edges that otherwise might dig into the corners of your toes.

Chafing

Chafing occurs when you sweat during the early stages of a run, then become dehydrated and stop sweating; the sweat dries, causing your skin to become salty. In turn, your skin becomes sticky and scratchy, which causes chafing. Deodorant can also become sticky and cause chafing.

To prevent chafing, try to stay dry by using a drying agent like talcum powder or starch, or continue to sweat by staying hydrated, which requires carrying water and drinking regularly on your run. If you do find that you have certain red and irritated spots on your body, perhaps under your arms or under the edges of your sport bra, be sure to apply a generous coat of Vaseline to the spots before heading out for your run. If left untreated, a chafed area can quickly turn into an open sore, which is even more painful and difficult to treat. You could also try a lubricant in areas that are predisposed to irritation, and one final suggestion is to wear breathable clothing that is snug but not tight.

Cold or flu

Over the course of your 26-week training program, it's likely that you will wake up one morning with the nagging feeling that you are coming down with a cold or flu bug. It happens to all of us, but what do you do when your training schedule has you running 5 miles? Should you rest, or persevere through the cold and hope for the best? Before you answer that question, check your symptoms. If you're feeling sick above the neck, such as having a sore throat or stuffy nose, a little running should be fine, but you might want to cut back and do only half the distance suggested in your program. Monitor yourself on your run—if you feel dizziness, have nausea, or experience excessive sweating, stop running. If you are feeling symptoms below the neck, such as muscle aches, chills, swollen glands, or a fever, that suggests a virus and increases the likelihood of dehydration. This can lead to more serious problems, so you should not run until you are completely recovered. If you are forced to take a few days off, it may take you a while to get back to where you were in your training, but before long you will be feeling like yourself again. Any more than a couple of days' rest shouldn't wreak havoc on your training plans, but if you have taken a week or more off, refer to chapter 4 for details on how to resume your distance-running program.

Rest

Sleep and rest are the building blocks of solid training. It's fine to occasionally miss a few hours of sleep, but not getting a sufficient amount on a regular basis will lead to problems. Your body's ability to recover diminishes with inadequate rest, so you need to make sleep a priority just like eating, drinking, and training.

Overtraining

Overtraining occurs when you run too frequently or too fast and with too little rest and recovery. The theory among those runners who overtrain often seems to be that if a specific amount of training is good, then more must be better. As a result, instead of running 20 miles (32 kilometers) a week these folks begin running 40 miles, then 50 miles, and maybe even 60 miles a week. Increased training might seem a good idea, especially if you are seeing an initial improvement in your fitness level and running ability, but the body has limits. It is especially important for beginning marathoners to realize that more is not better—marathon training in moderation is the best approach. But overtraining does happen, and it leaves runners at a much higher risk of injury and burnout. Some of the common signs and symptoms include:

- Ongoing muscle fatigue and soreness that does not dissipate
- Fatigue at the start of a run and difficulty meeting target pace goals
- Waning interest in training
- Unexplained weight loss
- Headaches
- Insomnia
- Inability to relax; twitchy and fidgety behavior

If you are suffering from a number of the above warning signs, take a few days off to rest and recover. Drink plenty of liquids, alter your diet if necessary, and if the symptoms don't go away within 2 or 3 days, be sure to check with your physician so that any potentially serious problems can be ruled out.

Staying Healthy

Overtraining is the most common cause of injury. Consistent training is definitely essential to making it to the marathon finish line. Sometimes, pushing through fatigue is needed in order to achieve your desired training effect, but it's important to get to know your body and to recognize when it's safer to back off and take a rest. In this respect, it's better to undertrain than to overtrain. Taking a break is not a sign of weakness. Rather, the opposite is true: it's smart training, because consistency over time is what's key.

Returning to Activity after Injury

Many exercisers endanger their immediate or future health by returning to action too soon. If you suffer an injury, keep in mind the following principles before returning to activity:

- Ensure pain-free range of motion in the previously injured area.
- Check that your strength, endurance, coordination, and speed of movement are equal to the uninjured side or back to pre-injury levels.
- Ensure that you are psychologically prepared to return and confident you will not be reinjured.

Alternative Training If You Become Injured

Injury rarely means complete rest is required. Try pool exercising or stationary cycling as a way to maintain

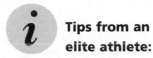

Tips from an elite athlete: Find some cold water

After a long run or hard workout, elite marathoner Art Boileau often heads to the ocean. With a large coffee in hand, he forces himself to wade in up to his waist and stand in the chilly water for 10 minutes while sipping his hot drink. He shivers through the whole experience, but the cold water reduces muscle swelling and inflammation. Great for speedy recovery!

your fitness level. You will keep your muscles in shape without the impact of running/walking. When you are ready to resume your run/walk program, remember to ease into it slowly. Your body needs time to readjust itself to exercising with full body weight.

What to Do If Forced to Miss Some Training

If you miss a session, don't fret—it happens to all of us once in a while. All you need is a good plan. The following are suggestions for returning to your training program in a safe and comfortable manner. Find the scenario that most closely resembles your situation, and follow the guidelines for returning to your marathon or half-marathon program after injury, illness, or unavoidable family or work demands.

Scenario 1: I'm not injured, but I missed almost 1 week of training

Return-to-activity guidelines

- If your program indicates that this should be an easy recovery week, you're in luck! Jump back in and resume training as though you haven't missed a beat.
- If your program indicates that this is not an easy recovery week, it's a little trickier, and you need to be cautious. For session 1, complete only the first half of the workout outlined for the current week. For sessions 2 and 3, complete workouts 2 and 3 from the previous week's training schedule. By doing two of the missed workouts from last week, you will be up to speed and ready to rejoin the current week's training program.

Scenario 2: I've missed more than 1 week, but not because of injury

One of the greatest benefits of walking and running is that you can do them anywhere, at any time, and all you need are a good pair of shoes and a program to follow. If you've missed more than 1 week of training but the interruption was not due to injury or illness, you may want to re-evaluate your commitment to your distance-running goal. In order to be successful in completing a marathon or half marathon in a safe and comfortable manner, you need to do your homework. This means following the suggested three sessions per week.

Return-to-activity guidelines

Week 1: Rejoin the program in the current week, but do only *half* the workout for each session.

Week 2: Continue with the program in the current week, but do only *three-quarters* of the workout for each session.

Week 3: Now you are ready to complete the *full* workout in the current week for each session.

And from now on, do your homework!

Scenario 3: I've missed up to 1 week because of injury

Cross training

If you have a nagging ache or pain that has been bothering you for a few days, and as a result you need to take a week off from the impact of running or walking, no worries! Cross training will maintain your fitness, and pool running is an effective way to duplicate your running and walking form.

In all cases, the very best scenario is to simply take the suggested workout of the day and transfer it directly to your cross-training activity. For example: if you were to do change-of-pace intervals of 2 minutes of brisk walking or jogging followed by 2 minutes of a slow and easy recovery, then you would jump into the deep end of a pool (or take to the cross-country trail or stationary bike) and do exactly those intervals, including the warm-up and cool-down. Remember, all the same principles apply: "brisk" means just slightly faster than a talking pace, and the rest is done at a nice, easy, talking pace.

Return-to-activity guidelines

Because you were sidelined by an injury, you need to be careful not do too much, too soon. It's important that you don't try to start back where you left off. Review the injury-awareness scale earlier in this chapter, and when you are ready, follow the suggestion in scenario 1.

Scenario 4: I've missed up to 2 weeks due to an injury

Cross training

See scenario 3. You need to make the effort to cross train for your three weekly sessions by transferring your marathon or half-marathon workout to pool running or a stationary bike, as described above. By doing this, you will maintain your fitness. You may feel a little awkward when you return to training on land (running or walking), but before you know it, these feelings will subside.

Return-to-activity guidelines

Because your injury likely was the result of impact, overuse, or pushing yourself too hard, it's important to carefully plan your return to activity. Review the injury-awareness scale earlier in this chapter. Avoid hard surfaces in favor of softer terrain such as grass or dirt trails when you resume training.

Weeks 1 and 2: Complete only *half* of what the workout suggests for each session.

Week 3: Complete only *three-quarters* of what the workout suggests for each session.

Week 4: Complete the *full* workout for each session, but only if your injury-awareness level has remained low.

Scenario 5: I've missed up to 3 weeks of the program due to injury

Cross training

See scenario 3. It's highly likely that you are feeling very frustrated. But have faith; if you make a sincere effort to cross train on your three sessions per week by transferring your workout to pool running or a stationary bike, as described in scenario 3, you can maintain your fitness. Honest. You will feel awkward when you resume training on land, but that won't last. It's worth being cautious in order to avoid reinjuring yourself. If there is not enough time to recover before your event, you may have to reassess your goals.

Scenario 6: I've missed more than 3 weeks of the program

At this point your situation must be assessed individually. You may have to rethink your running goal, or choose an event at a later date and plan your training program accordingly.

Final Preparations

THIS IS IT, THE DAY YOU HAVE BEEN PREPARING FOR. Chances are you are in the best physical condition ever. First-time marathoners often feel a significant level of anxiety in the week leading up to their half or full marathon. Try to relax. Some nervousness is normal, but you want to do as much as you can to calm yourself. Anxiety takes energy, and the last thing we want is for you to be fatigued on your big day.

Before a marathon, many athletes like to scope out the course and get a feel for the environment they will be running in. You can drive it, or if you're doing a half marathon, you could cycle or even run part of the course. If you're a first-timer, you might want to run only part of the route; you don't want to tire yourself out for race day. Many people find that getting a mental picture of the course helps them to understand the terrain and visualize what race day will be like. It's also good to know what kind of surface you'll be running on, whether it's pavement or gravel. The more you know about what your race will look like, the more relaxed and ready you will be on the morning of your event.

Taper Your Training

Tapering is a gradual reduction in training volume and intensity prior to a race. For the body to be rested and ready to complete a distance event, it needs time to recover from the weeks and months of marathon training. Too often runners want to train right up to the marathon, but everyone—even the most seasoned marathoner—needs time to recover after all the months of hard training. The extra rest allows damaged muscles to heal. Our training programs have you reducing the length of your long runs in the 3-week period leading up to your race. In the final days before it you are hardly running, doing so only to reduce nervousness and loosen up your muscles and joints before the big event.

Plan for Your Race Day

You have worked long and hard to prepare for your half or full marathon. You don't want to leave anything to chance at this point in the game. A little bit of planning for race day will make all the difference in how you enjoy the experience. Here are some simple guidelines for event preparation:

- Rest in the last few days before the event. Squeezing in more training at the last minute will not get you any fitter. Plan to get an optimal amount of sleep during the final 72 hours.
- Keep your daily routines as normal as possible—this is not the time to try something new!
- Check the weather forecast the day before the race and plan accordingly. Consider what you will wear during the run, as well as what you will wear after it.

- Pack your bag and pin your number on your shirt the night before. Items to consider (depending on the time of year): a complete change of clothes, extra shoes, a hat, gloves, toilet paper (you'd be surprised how often it's needed), petroleum jelly, a towel, a rain jacket, and a bottle of water.

- Be sure to drink plenty of water—2 to 3 glasses, 1 to 2 hours before the start. (Also, don't forget to drink water at the aid stations along the running route.)

Jen

Jen was 25 and in her second year of nursing when she decided to train for the Portland Marathon. She had done several 10-kilometer (6-mile) races and three half marathons in the past couple of years and felt confident that with a good training program she would be able to run/walk 26.2 miles (42 kilometers) on race day. She was meticulous with her preparation, following a 6-month marathon program and altering her diet and sleep habits to coincide with her training. But in the days leading up to race day, she was surprised at the level of anxiety she felt whenever she thought about the event. At first, it was just some mild tension, similar to what she had experienced before previous races, but 2 days before race day she was riddled with anxiety. She questioned whether her body would allow her to travel the distance. Had she trained enough? Was she starting to feel the onset of a cold or flu?

On the morning of the race, Jen had basically talked herself out of doing the marathon until a friend, who was sort of a running mentor, encouraged her to ignore these concerns and focus on all the hard work she had done. She told her that once she was a few miles into the race, she would begin to relax. Her friend was right. After mile 2, Jen was calm and quickly relaxed into a good pattern of walk/running that easily carried her to the finish. In the days following the race, she again spoke with her running mentor about her anxiety and bad nerves leading up to the race and was relieved to learn that all of her pre-race jitters were perfectly normal. Next time, Jen will be mentally prepared to deal with the fear and extreme nervousness that comes with the marathon.

Once the gun goes off

- Don't start out too fast. The first few miles should feel easy.
- Do the talk test. If you're having difficulty speaking four or five consecutive sentences, you're going too fast and need to back off. You should not be winded or breathing hard at all in the first 10 to 15 miles (16 to 24 kilometers) of your marathon.
- Walking through the aid stations makes it easier to consume your water or food supplements, and it gives you a chance to rest your legs.
- During the race, try to take in as much of the event as you can. You will be nervous, but if you smile and look around, it will help you to relax and enjoy the moment. After all, it's your big day, and you want to drink it all in!

- Plan a little extra time for pre-race bathroom visits. Anxiety will likely necessitate these, and lineups for the washrooms can be quite long!
- When driving to the race, give yourself plenty of time to park, visit the restroom, and warm up.
- Warm up properly. Although there is no guarantee this will prevent injuries, a combination of light jogging and easy stretching prior to the start will increase your heart rate and help loosen joints and muscles, preparing your body for the activity ahead.
- Try to keep as warm and dry as possible before the start of the race.
- Don't wear new gear such as shoes, socks, or a sport bra, and never experiment with new food or drinks the day prior to or on the morning of your event.

Anticipating Your Finishing Time

A runner who has been training regularly three or four times a week can often predict his or her marathon time by multiplying a recent half-marathon time in minutes by 2 and adding 10 minutes. Beginners should add an additional 10 minutes to be safe. If a well-trained person is preparing for a half marathon, he or she usually multiplies a recent 10-kilometer time in minutes by 2 and adds 5 to 7 minutes. Beginners should add a further 5 minutes to be safe.

There are numerous on-line charts that help you to predict your time based on shorter-distance events such as a 5- or 10-kilometer race. It might be difficult, but try not to worry about your time. First-timers should focus more on finishing than on finishing fast.

What is a reasonable length of time to run a marathon?

There is no such thing as a reasonable time to run a marathon. Male elite runners finish in and around 2 hours; top female runners cross the finish line in about 2 hours and 20 minutes. Still, it is not uncommon for people to walk/run the half marathon in 2 to 3 hours and the full marathon in 5 to 6 hours.

The Mental Challenges of Race Day

It is normal for you to feel nervous in the days leading up to your event. On race-day morning, you may even find you're asking yourself, "Why do I want to attempt such a monstrous task?" Relax—these are what is referred to as pre-race jitters. Most runners, even the elite, experience a certain level of anxiety before an event. How you handle it is up to you. Try reminding yourself of all the hard work you have put into preparing for your event. If you have followed the training program to the best of your ability, you will have the fitness level required to complete the distance. Consider all of the long runs you have done in the lead-up to this distance; these runs have prepared you not only physically but also mentally for many of the challenges you will face on race day.

Things will be similar in many ways on race day, but they will also be quite different. After all your months of training, you will be rested and ready. Chances are you will be incredibly motivated once you are among the hordes of other runners and the spectators who will be cheering you to the finish. You will be pleasantly surprised at the friendly and welcoming atmosphere of your event. Regardless of whether you're an elite runner or a beginner, there is nothing like the excitement of the start line and the exhilaration of the finish. Once the gun goes off to signal the start, you will find that after a couple of miles all of your nervousness has disappeared.

Remembering to be positive

In chapter 6 we talked about the impact self-talk can have on your running experience. Before your event, try to take some time to think about your ability to use positive self-talk. If you haven't already done so, create a list of statements you can use during your event to bolster your self-confidence as well as your mood and overall view of the experience. You are going to have periods during the race when you'll experience discouraging thoughts. By having a list of statements to review, you can more easily bypass these negative thoughts. The statements need to mean something to you. Motivation is different for each individual. The words that motivate or inspire your training partner might not help you, so give it some thought and begin making a list. Here are a few statements to consider:

- I have not put pressure on myself.
- I'm going to enjoy this.
- I'll start very slowly.
- This is an amazing event.
- Everyone is so strong and so am I.
- I'm a runner.
- Strong and smooth is the way to go.

- I started slowly, so I can definitely make it to the finish.
- I ran this far on my training run, so I can do it again today.
- I love myself, and I respect myself—I can do this for me.
- I'm doing this for me and only me.

Pacing

During your event, don't forget to pace yourself. After all, it's a long way to the finish line. It's easy to get caught up in the excitement, and many first-timers start out too fast, only to pay for it later with early muscle fatigue or cramps that could easily have been avoided. Once you start running, check in with yourself by doing the talk test. You should be able to speak four or five consecutive sentences without getting winded. If this isn't the case, you need to back off and run slower.

Hitting the Wall

"Hitting the wall" is a common phrase used by marathon runners when referring to a point in a race when they run out of energy. Basically, you have hit the wall when your fuel supply no longer meets your energy demands. The runner who hits the wall has two choices: drop out of the race, or slow down and endure the discomfort of tight and burning muscles until the finish line is reached.

A marathon expert and author, Jeff Galloway, says approximately 40 percent of all non-elite marathon runners have hit the wall. The good news is that this can easily be avoided with good pre-race nutrition and by proper hydration and suitable nutrition throughout the race.

Bonking

The body's stored carbohydrate supply (glycogen) is limited. Says sport dietitian Dallas Parsons, "It is only able to provide the body with enough fuel for 1 to 2 hours of moderate-intensity exercise." Once the body uses the carbohydrate or glycogen stores, it begins a process that is commonly referred to in athletic circles as bonking.

One of the first signs of bonking comes when you have difficulty putting one foot in front of the other because the muscles in your legs have run out of glycogen. At this point, you will not have any psychological side effects. You can easily minimize the physical effects by immediately taking in a source of carbohydrates (30 grams, or about an ounce) such as a gel or sport drink and continuing to refuel for the duration of your event. If bonking is left untreated, however, you will continue on a downward slope. In addition to the muscles in your legs running out of fuel, your brain will begin to lack a supply of glucose. At this stage runners experience a myriad of different symptoms ranging from dizziness to confusion to collapse, which can lead to a dangerous condition requiring medical attention.

You can easily avoid any stage of glycogen depletion or bonking by starting out your run properly fueled from a carb-rich meal or snack at least 2 hours prior to running. Consuming a carbohydrate source during runs lasting longer than 90 minutes will also reduce the chances of bonking. If you train after work, be sure to have a substantial snack with 50 to 100 grams of carbohydrate beforehand. If you train early in the morning and don't have time for a full breakfast, try to have some quick carbs like toast and jelly, a sport drink, or gel with water before you begin your run. If you're planning to run longer than 60 minutes in the morning, take along a carb snack such as an energy bar. You have fasted overnight and already depleted your carbohydrate stores.

Common Questions

What should I eat the night before my event?

There aren't any magic meals to guarantee a great race, but here are some suggestions to help plan your pre-race meal.

- Try to eat dinner between 5:00 and 7:00 PM to allow your body time to digest your food before bed.
- During your event you will burn primarily carbohydrates. Try a pasta dish with a tomato-and-meat sauce, or a meat stir-fry with a light dressing. Vegetarians should remember to include some form of protein like tofu or beans.
- Avoid cream sauces and soups. Use fats such as oils, margarine, and dressings sparingly.
- Include some whole grain bread and a salad with a light vinaigrette dressing.

- Keep alcohol to a minimum, and don't forget your usual 6 to 8 glasses of non-caffeinated drinks such as juice, milk, sport drink, and water the day before the race.
- If you want dessert, fruit, low-fat yogurt, or a home-baked oatmeal cookie are good choices.

What should I have for my race-day breakfast?

- Eat a couple of hours before you begin your warm-up, and keep it simple: granola cereal is a good choice, but stay away from bran.
- Have some whole grain toast with jam or honey. Fruit is good, especially bananas. Clear juices are fine.
- A small amount of coffee or tea shouldn't be a problem.

What if I get a cold before the race?

- If it happens the week before, with luck you can manage your symptoms and be ready for race day.
- Rest, drink plenty of fluids, coupled with ibuprofen as directed on the bottle and perhaps some extra vitamin C.
- Don't worry about trying to follow your marathon program. In one week you will not lose any fitness, and you're better off taking care of yourself and saving your energy for race day.
- Fresh air is always a good idea. A short walk followed by a few stretches is a great way to keep you limber, and, when you're sick, it's good for your spirits!
- If you're very sick, consult your family physician and please make the right decision. You can always find another marathon event in the next few weeks when

you're feeling better. Revisit chapter 9 for a more detailed description of what to do if you find yourself with a cold or flu bug during your training program.

Should I warm up before the race?

- Yes. As during your workouts, you need to warm up before the main event.
- About 30 minutes before the race starts, warm up for 5 or 10 minutes by walking or jogging. One idea is to use your warm-up jog as your mode of travel to the start area from where you've parked your car or disembarked from the bus.
- You'll have to weave your way through the crowds to your start "wave," but try to stay limber by doing some dynamic active stretches: arm circles, trunk circles, knee lifts, and light jogging on the spot. Try to keep moving until the start gun goes.

What do I need to do the night before the race?

- Organize yourself for race day, anticipating all types of weather. Preparing now will allow you to have a good night's rest and avoid last-minute organizing in the morning.
- Ensure you have at the ready your race number, timing chip (laced into your shoes—most events these days use a computer chip to keep track of participants and ensure accurate record keeping for everyone), shorts or tights, socks, jacket, hat for rain or sun, sunscreen, and a watch. Take a set of dry clothing and shoes for afterward.

- Review other items including a water bottle and perhaps a water bottle pack, cell phone, and money for a taxi or whatever other need might present itself.

- If you're driving or taking a run-team bus, it's easy to take all your gear permutations with you and simply leave the extras behind when you go to the start line. If you're traveling on public transport, you'll have to be more selective and manage your gear in a small knapsack if you don't have an option of leaving it with a support person at the event.

How much should I drink before and during the race?

- Your body should already be well hydrated before your event. To suddenly start drinking a lot of water is not a good idea.

- Continually sipping small amounts of water throughout the day and every day is the best plan, so if that's not your usual habit, it's okay to start in the week before the race.

- Try to drink 6 to 8 glasses of water a day, and if you are used to carrying a water bottle when you train, then carry one during the event.

- There will be water stations set up along the course, and if you were to stop and take water at each one you would be adequately hydrated throughout the event.

What last-minute checks should I make?

- At the marathon or half-marathon event, when the start gun is moments away, make sure your laces are double-knotted, your number is pinned on comfortably, and your stopwatch timer is set to zero. Take a little sip of water. Wish yourself and those around you good luck, and keep moving in whatever space you have until you hear the gun and you're able to make a start.

- If this is your first marathon or half-marathon event, it isn't important that you start at the front. You might even want to start toward the back of the pack. Regardless of where you are at the start, your time will be properly recorded because your timing chip is activated only when you cross the start line.

How do I relax the night before and at the start line?

- It's hard to relax when you're really excited about something, but you can seek comfort in the fact that the night before the event, the work is done, and there's really nothing more you can do other than put your feet up and do something you enjoy.
- Have your optimal pre-event dinner, organize your gear, and kick back and relax with family and/or friends.
- Watching movies or reading are pleasant distractions, as are any other mellow, easygoing activities.

Can I set time goals for the marathon or half marathon?

- Some of you will already have a specific, realistic goal in mind for your event finish time. Some of you will be less specific, more intrinsic, with a goal focused more on participation and safely and comfortably completing the distance.

- If you want to set a time goal, refer to the Event-Day Pace Chart on page 83 to estimate your finishing time. By timing how long it takes you to run a mile, you can calculate your approximate race-day finish time. Many beginners add 10 or 15 minutes to this time just to be safe. If nothing else, your approximate goal time gives your family and friends an estimation of when they should meet you at the finish line!

After the Finish Line

11

YOU DID IT! THIS IS A TRULY AMAZING ACCOMPLISHMENT. You persevered and achieved a goal most people wouldn't even dare to dream about. Congratulations—you are now an official member of the marathoners' club. No doubt you are feeling pretty good.

Whether you're an elite athlete or a first-time marathoner, the moment your foot touches the finish line the feelings of euphoria are the same. The marathon is a race of champions. It is a race that demands great physical endurance, as well as mental and emotional strength. From the initial feelings of joy and jubilation to stiff muscles and overall fatigue to finding your next fitness goal, this chapter answers most of the commonly asked post-race questions.

Crossing the Finish Line

You will feel tremendous excitement and exhilaration as you run across the finish line. Drink in these feelings, and take the time to enjoy your accomplishment. You earned it. Don't downplay your achievement; you are amazing. Enjoy the limelight, and have fun sharing your experience with friends, family, and colleagues. For most people, completing a half or full marathon is one of their biggest lifetime feats.

It's important to know that you're also going to feel pretty exhausted. You can anticipate a few aches and pains, but most of your physical discomfort will be minimized by your overwhelming mental high. A proper post-event plan like the one below will help to make your initial recovery a little easier:

- Within 45 minutes of finishing, eat or drink a snack of 200 to 500 calories. It's a good idea to walk for at least 10 minutes while you drink and eat, to cool down. Finish off with some light stretching.
- If it's been raining or is a cold day, immediately change into warm and dry clothing.
- If it's been a hot day, consume a fluid-replacement drink that contains sodium.
- Take care of any blisters that developed during your event.
- If you can, immerse your legs in a cold bath as soon as possible following your finish.
- Later in the day, try to go for a short walk, and continue to drink fluids every hour.
- Pay close attention to your hydration in the 24 to 48 hours after your event. If your urine is dark or tea-colored, check with your physician to make sure everything is okay.
- In the day following the race, walk for 30 to 60 minutes at a leisurely pace to help stretch your muscles.

A need for rest

After first-timers complete a half or full marathon, they experience a great deal of personal satisfaction and commonly want to resume training immediately.

Although completing this type of distance event is very motivating, it's important to be extremely cautious in the following days and weeks.

Training for and completing distance races puts major strain on the body and results in small tears in the muscular tissue. This is normal. These small tears require a significant amount of time to heal and regenerate. It would be dangerous and potentially harmful to resume any kind of intense training immediately following your event.

"Runners who complete a half or full marathon need to take a commonsense approach in their return to running," says Louisiana sport medicine physician Dr. Bryan Barootes. By doing so, they drastically reduce the likelihood of incurring an injury.

After the Marathon

In the hours following the marathon, you will likely have trouble getting up from a chair or walking down stairs, and you will feel a general sense of fatigue and soreness in the hips and joints. "There are numerous variables affecting how people will feel post-marathon, in terms of what they've eaten during the marathon and how much they drank," says Dr. Barootes. "Weather conditions are also an influencing factor. If, for example, temperatures were high and you were on the course for 6 hours, you may have experienced slight heat exhaustion or dehydration that would require extra recovery time."

How to recover

Dr. Barootes uses a "10 percent rule" to gauge marathon and half-marathon recovery. "Every day following the marathon, runners should feel a 10 percent improvement in how they feel. A week after, your stiffness should be gone, and at the end of the second week most people will feel like they're back to normal." This is not an exact science, so setting concrete parameters is not wise. For example, runners who complete a half marathon will not necessarily feel half as tired or be half as sore as full-marathoners. In most cases, half-marathoners will have walked/run at a speed faster than they would maintain over 26.2 miles (42 kilometers). This means they worked at a higher intensity over 13.1 miles (21 kilometers) than full-marathoners did over 26.2, which is why the recovery time for the two events is similar.

The important factor to remember is to be conservative in your recovery and recognize that it depends on the individual. It might, for example, take your friend 7 days to rid himself of muscle stiffness, but it might take you 22 days. What's key is that you give yourself the right amount of time to fully recover.

Easing back into an exercise program

Once the excitement of completing your event has worn off, you may feel an emotional dip. It's not uncommon for athletes to experience a small degree of post-event depression after completing a half or full marathon. This can be attributed to achieving a goal that you have spent a great deal of time and energy to accomplish. Your routine of the past 4 to 6 months has been thrown off, and you now feel a void in your life. When this happens, it's common to feel a little down. Dr. Barootes says the emotional low may persist until you get back into your running, start a new activity, or set another goal for yourself.

It's safe to resume some exercise once you start feeling like yourself again. "You're ready for some moderate exercise once you are no longer experiencing any pain in your everyday activities, like walking up and down stairs," Dr. Barootes says. He encourages athletes to start with non-strenuous activities such as walking, cycling, or swimming. Moderation is the key—you don't want to overdo it, for example risking injury with a long bike ride two weeks after completing a marathon.

Setting Your Next Goal

Now that you've completed a half or full marathon you will likely think of yourself as a different person. You have taken yourself to a new level of fitness and probably given your self-confidence a boost as well. You know that if you set your mind to something, you can achieve it. If you have trained with others, you will have made new friends outside your traditional circle. But once the race is over, you may find yourself asking, "Now what?"

From a physiological standpoint, your successful completion of the program brings you both good news and bad. The good news is that the cardiovascular (heart and lungs) fitness you have worked so patiently to develop over the past 4 to 6 months is relatively easy to maintain. All you have to do is carry on doing what you have been doing—exercise aerobically three times a week for 30 to 40 minutes. You do not have to perpetually push yourself further. If, however, you want to continue to improve your fitness level, you're going to have to continue challenging your body. One way to do this is to train to run a marathon or half marathon at a faster pace. This might involve, for example, some speed training or hill work that focuses on making you stronger and faster. There is a lot of information on speed training on-line.

The bad news is that if you've thought of the completion of your training program as the end of the road, the fitness you have worked so hard to attain will slowly seep away, like water into sand. After a few months, it will be vastly diminished. You may find it unfair that you worked so hard and yet can't rest on your laurels for a while, but that's the way it is. Your body will return to the state it was in before you started the program.

Some people don't mind. They may have taken on the program simply to see if they could do it, or because a friend challenged them. Sometimes these people drift away from fitness altogether and never come back. It's a personal choice—though not a very healthy one.

Other people find that when they get to the end of the program and don't have a schedule to follow, their motivation slips out the door. It's not so much a choice: they're out of shape again.

If this happens to you, or if a life event—sickness in the family, say, or a crisis at work—prevents you from maintaining your current level of fitness, you can always start again. It isn't as bad as it sounds. You already know that in your hand you have both the prescription and the cure. Many people who let their fitness slide after completing a half- or full-marathon program eventually become unhappy about huffing and puffing like an old steam locomotive every time they have to sprint for the bus, and they return to the program a few or even many months later. It is infinitely better to start again than it is to quit for good.

What next?

You may decide that you want to return to running but need time to settle on your next goal. That goal doesn't have to be marathon focused. You may want to improve your speed and train for a 5- or 10-kilometer (3- or 6-mile) event. You might give some thought to completing a triathlon. Taking a few weeks off after your marathon or half marathon will help you to recover, but once you're feeling yourself, ease back into your active lifestyle; your fitness level will still be great. Even if you take months to return to running, be gentle with yourself. Remember that once you get into a regular running program, it won't be long before you begin to feel like the marathon or half-marathon runner that you are.

If you're not sure what to do next for your running program, and you don't want to begin training for another half or full marathon, there are a number of approaches to staying in top form. You can simply commit to running three 30- to 40-minute sessions a week, which should be relatively easy because your body is already programmed to run even more than this. You can adjust the time training to suit your schedule.

You may find you want to continue with one longer run on the weekend; this might be an ideal opportunity to meet up with your former marathon-training partners. Many runners continue to meet after completing their

Nancy

Nancy, 48, is a stay-at-home mom with four children between the ages of 10 and 15. Now that the girls are getting a little older, Nancy has more time to explore her own hobbies and passions. At first she considered volunteering for a few hours a week with a women's shelter, but then a friend suggested she explore her running potential and possibly train for a marathon. Nancy thought her friend was crazy. After all, it would take time to train, which would mean time away from her responsibilities at home. Her husband worked long hours so that she could stay at home, and she truly appreciated the opportunity to be a hands-on mom, but the idea of doing something completely for herself was exciting.

After some encouragement from her marathoning girlfriends, Nancy broached with her family the subject of her training for a marathon. To her surprise, the entire family started to cheer. Her husband, Seth, was especially excited. Everyone seemed to think she needed to get out of the house and explore the world beyond homemaking. She started to research different marathon programs and eventually decided to join a training group at her local community center. She wasn't sure about the idea of running in a group, but she decided she would benefit from training with others and learning from an experienced run leader.

Nancy was surprised at how nervous she was on the morning of her first group run. Her family surprised her with a new running top for her first marathon-training session. Part of her wanted to drop out of the program and train on her own, but her family would be disappointed, so she forced herself to go to the initial workout. After the first couple of training runs, she became comfortable with the group and enjoyed listening to the chatter around her. Before long she was able to chat with some of the others in the group while running, and over the months of training she was amazed at how much she looked forward to her group runs. She had even started to meet a couple of the other women for runs during the week. She now finds the upcoming marathon exciting, and she doesn't know how she would have trained over the months had it not been for her run group.

event because the experience of training for and completing a race is a bonding encounter that cannot be easily replicated.

If you find your motivation slipping away, sign up for one of the many running and walking events in your community. There are runners everywhere these days, and most of them love getting together. The events they attend are partly a way to gauge progress and partly a way to socialize. Your local running-shoe store or community center will likely have a schedule of such events. As well, walking clubs abound, and their weekly activities are often listed in local newspapers.

If you complete a half or full marathon and decide that running isn't for you, don't despair. Running isn't for everyone, which is probably a good thing, because if it were, some running paths would get very crowded. Still, not loving to run shouldn't mean retreating to the sofa and the television remote control. As discussed in chapter 7, there are all kinds of other enjoyable aerobic activities. Cycling, swimming, cross-country skiing, and hiking are excellent alternatives to running, as are in-line skating, kayaking, aerobics to music, walking, or even just putting in some time on the stair climber at your local gym.

When approaching any sport, remember the three rules of exercise—moderation, consistency, and rest—and don't expect to be an expert right away. Each sport requires unique skills, and it will take you a while to acquire them. Each time you take up a new activity, you'll find there are as many comfort-zone barriers to cross as you are willing to take on. As well, you will

Take a break from running

- Once you're recovered from your distance event, resume some light exercise for a few weeks before getting back into a running program. Most people need at least 3 weeks to fully recover from a marathon or half marathon.
- When you are ready to run, start with three easy 30-minute outings.
- Join a running or walking club.
- Sign up for running or walking events. Check your local running-shoe store or community center for details.
- Continue to keep an exercise/activity log to record your workouts.
- Try other activities. Cycling, swimming, and hiking are just a few of the numerous, excellent alternatives to running.
- If you've just completed the marathon and are psyched for another, it's advisable to wait 4 to 6 months. It's wise to do no more than 2 or 3 marathons per year. Half-marathoners should wait 2 or 3 months before attempting the next one.

invariably reach plateaus of competence that only patience and practice will take you beyond. If you're having trouble progressing, take lessons, or seek assistance from a more experienced participant; every sport has a dedicated core of enthusiasts who are glad to help newcomers.

Sarah and Bill

Sarah had been a regular runner for years, and when she began dating Bill, they started to join each other for the odd run. Bill, a great all-round athlete, was thrilled to have met a woman who shared his passion for fitness. Given his busy teaching schedule and his work to finish his doctoral dissertation, he found it was great to get in a workout and have time with Sarah.

Sarah and Bill continued dating and eventually moved in together. Over the years, Bill often remarked that he felt most connected with her when they shared regular runs. "Sometimes we don't even speak, we just enjoy exploring the nearby trails. And there's something romantic about sharing the calmness of the early morning light. We always return from our runs happier, more at peace with the world and with each other. For both of us, running is truly a gift."

Three years after the couple met, Bill proposed to Sarah and at the same time suggested they run a marathon together in celebration of their partnership. Sarah was thrilled about their engagement and touched by Bill's marathon idea. In the months of training leading up to the marathon, she was increasingly concerned that as the faster runner he would find her slower pace tedious during the later stages of the race. But he assured her the pace would be fine, and on race day he showed no impatience. At mile 20, when Sarah's calf muscle started to spasm, Bill helped with stretching suggestions, and he massaged her leg. The two finished the marathon together, and they have a finishing photo to show for their joint achievement.

Sarah didn't reach her sub-3:10 marathon time goal, but it didn't matter. "We were both amazed that after running 26.2 miles together, we were still smiling and joking with each other. Bill was so supportive; I look forward to a future race where I can somehow do the same for him!"

Appendix A

Stretching Exercises

Here are some stretches for the major muscle groups used in running and walking. Use them as a guide to building your own routine. It's a good idea to work systematically from the calves up to the shoulders (or vice versa).

Before stretching, always start with 5 to 10 minutes of jogging on the spot, or slow and easy running, to warm your muscles. Then move into your pre-training stretching exercises. Hold each position (no bouncing) for approximately 30 seconds. Your stretching routine should take no more than 10 to 12 minutes.

After your workout, use the same stretches to cool down. If you wish to work on increasing your flexibility, hold the stretches for longer—anywhere from 30 seconds to 3 minutes—and repeat each stretch 2 to 3 times. Pay particular attention to the areas that you feel are the tightest; in runners, these are usually the lower back, hamstrings, and calves.

Calf

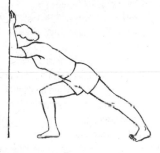

1. Stand facing a wall, an arm's length plus 6 inches (15 centimeters) away.
2. Place your right foot forward, halfway to the wall, and bend your right knee while keeping your left leg straight.
3. Lean into the wall, pushing your left heel into the floor while keeping your head, neck, spine, pelvis, and left leg in a straight line.
4. Hold the stretch for 30 seconds and relax.
5. Repeat, starting with your left leg forward.

Hamstring

This exercise requires a doorway.

1. Lie flat on your back, through a doorway, positioning your hips slightly in front of the door frame, with the inside of your lower right thigh against one side of the frame.
2. Keeping your right leg straight and flat on the floor, exhale and raise your left leg until your heel rests against the door frame. Do not bend your left knee.
3. Hold the stretch for 30 seconds and relax.
4. To increase the stretch, slide your buttocks closer to the door frame, or lift the leg away from the frame to create a right angle.
5. Repeat with your right leg raised.

Iliotibial Band

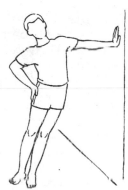

1. Stand with your left side toward a wall, an arm's length away, feet together.
2. Extend your left arm sideways at shoulder height so the flat of your hand is against the wall and you are leaning toward it.
3. Exhale, and push your left hip in toward the wall until you feel the stretch down the outside of your left hip/thigh.
4. Hold the stretch for 30 seconds and relax.
5. Repeat on the right side.

Quadriceps

Avoid this exercise if it causes pain in the knee joint.

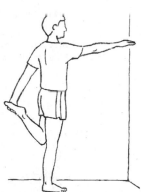

1. Stand tall, facing a wall, an arm's length away; place your right hand against the wall for balance and support.
2. Bend your left leg at the knee and raise the foot behind you until you can grasp it with your left hand.
3. Slightly bend your right leg at the knee and be sure to keep your lower back straight.
4. Keeping the knees together, pull your left heel toward your buttock.
5. Hold the stretch for 30 seconds and relax.
6. Repeat with your right leg.

Groin

1. Sit upright on the floor, with your back against a wall.
2. Bend your knees up, then let them fall to the sides, with the soles of your feet facing each other.
3. Grasp your ankles with both hands and pull your heels toward your buttocks.
4. Rest your elbows on the inside of your thighs.
5. Slowly push your knees toward the floor until you feel the stretch in your groin.
6. Hold the stretch for 30 seconds and relax.

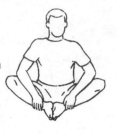

Hip Flexor

For those who are unable to kneel, this exercise can be done while sitting on the edge of a chair and assuming the same position as illustrated but without the knee touching the ground.

1. Stand with your feet hip-width apart.
2. Flexing your right knee, slowly lower your body toward the ground, finishing with your left knee touching the floor and your right heel flat on the floor.
3. Rest your hands just above the right knee, and keep that knee bent at no more than a right angle.
4. For some, getting into this position will be enough. If you wish to increase the stretch, exhale while pushing your left hip forward and increasing the stretch on the left side.
5. Hold the stretch for 30 seconds and relax.
6. Repeat with your left foot forward.

Gluteal

1. Lie flat on your back with your legs straight and arms out to the sides.

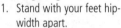

2. Bend the left knee and raise it toward your chest, grasping your knee or thigh with your right hand.
3. Keep your head, shoulders, and elbows flat on the floor.
4. Exhale as you pull your knee across your body toward the floor.
5. Hold the stretch for 30 seconds and relax.
6. For a deeper stretch, straighten the top leg.
7. Repeat with the right leg.

Lower Back

1. Lie flat on your back with your knees bent to form a right angle and your arms out to the sides.
2. Exhale, and slowly lower both knees to the left side.
3. Keep your elbows, head, and shoulders flat on the floor.
4. Hold the stretch for 30 seconds and relax.
5. Repeat on the right side.

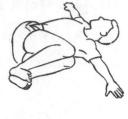

Lower Back

1. Lie flat on your back with your legs straight out.
2. Bend your knees and slide your heels toward your buttocks.
3. Using both hands, grasp behind your knees. (It's not important to keep your knees together—they should be comfortable.)
4. Exhale, pulling your knees toward your chest and slowly lifting your hips from the floor, while keeping your head and shoulders on the floor.
5. Hold the stretch for 30 seconds and relax.

Chest and Shoulder Stretch

1. Stand with your right arm straight and your right hand pressed against a wall behind you.
2. Walk your feet around so the toes point away from the wall.
3. With your right hand still resting against the wall, twist your hips and shoulders away from the wall, until you feel a slight stretch in the chest and shoulder.
4. Hold the stretch for 30 seconds and relax.
5. Repeat with left arm.

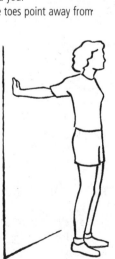

Appendix B

Link to Web site: http://www.csep.ca/pdfs/par-q.pdf

Physical Activity Readiness
Questionnaire - PAR-Q
(revised 2002)

PAR-Q & YOU

(A Questionnaire for People Aged 15 to 69)

Regular physical activity is fun and healthy, and increasingly more people are starting to become more active every day. Being more active is very safe for most people. However, some people should check with their doctor before they start becoming much more physically active.

If you are planning to become much more physically active than you are now, start by answering the seven questions in the box below. If you are between the ages of 15 and 69, the PAR-Q will tell you if you should check with your doctor before you start. If you are over 69 years of age, and you are not used to being very active, check with your doctor.

Common sense is your best guide when you answer these questions. Please read the questions carefully and answer each one honestly: check YES or NO.

YES	NO		
☐	☐	1.	Has your doctor ever said that you have a heart condition <u>and</u> that you should only do physical activity recommended by a doctor?
☐	☐	2.	Do you feel pain in your chest when you do physical activity?
☐	☐	3.	In the past month, have you had chest pain when you were not doing physical activity?
☐	☐	4.	Do you lose your balance because of dizziness or do you ever lose consciousness?
☐	☐	5.	Do you have a bone or joint problem (for example, back, knee or hip) that could be made worse by a change in your physical activity?
☐	☐	6.	Is your doctor currently prescribing drugs (for example, water pills) for your blood pressure or heart condition?
☐	☐	7.	Do you know of <u>any other reason</u> why you should not do physical activity?

If you answered

YES to one or more questions

Talk with your doctor by phone or in person BEFORE you start becoming much more physically active or BEFORE you have a fitness appraisal. Tell your doctor about the PAR-Q and which questions you answered YES.

- You may be able to do any activity you want — as long as you start slowly and build up gradually. Or, you may need to restrict your activities to those which are safe for you. Talk with your doctor about the kinds of activities you wish to participate in and follow his/her advice.
- Find out which community programs are safe and helpful for you.

NO to all questions

If you answered NO honestly to all PAR-Q questions, you can be reasonably sure that you can:
- start becoming much more physically active — begin slowly and build up gradually. This is the safest and easiest way to go.
- take part in a fitness appraisal — this is an excellent way to determine your basic fitness so that you can plan the best way for you to live actively. It is also highly recommended that you have your blood pressure evaluated. If your reading is over 144/94, talk with your doctor before you start becoming much more physically active.

DELAY BECOMING MUCH MORE ACTIVE:
- if you are not feeling well because of a temporary illness such as a cold or a fever — wait until you feel better; or
- if you are or may be pregnant — talk to your doctor before you start becoming more active.

PLEASE NOTE: If your health changes so that you then answer YES to any of the above questions, tell your fitness or health professional. Ask whether you should change your physical activity plan.

Informed Use of the PAR-Q: The Canadian Society for Exercise Physiology, Health Canada, and their agents assume no liability for persons who undertake physical activity, and if in doubt after completing this questionnaire, consult your doctor prior to physical activity.

No changes permitted. You are encouraged to photocopy the PAR-Q but only if you use the entire form.

NOTE: If the PAR-Q is being given to a person before he or she participates in a physical activity program or a fitness appraisal, this section may be used for legal or administrative purposes.

"I have read, understood and completed this questionnaire. Any questions I had were answered to my full satisfaction."

NAME _____

SIGNATURE _____ DATE _____

SIGNATURE OF PARENT _____ WITNESS _____
or GUARDIAN (for participants under the age of majority)

Note: This physical activity clearance is valid for a maximum of 12 months from the date it is completed and becomes invalid if your condition changes so that you would answer YES to any of the seven questions.

CSEP SCPE © Canadian Society for Exercise Physiology   Supported by: 🍁 Health Santé Canada Canada

continued on other side...

Printed by permission of the Canadian Society for Exercise Physiology

Appendix C

Zero to Marathon or Half Marathon in 26 Weeks

Pattern	Mon.	Tues.	Wed.	Thurs.	Fri.	Sat. Long-Run Day	Sun.
Week 1 We've begun! Comfortable	Off	Warm-up: Shuffle 5 min. Shuffle 1 min. Walk 2 min. Do this 8 times Cool-down: Walk 5 min. **Total time: 34 min.**	Off	Warm-up: Walk 5 min. Shuffle 1 min. Walk 2 min. Do this 6 times Cool-down: Walk 5 min. **Total time: 28 min.**	Optional cross training day	**Half Marathon:** Warm-up: Walk 5 min. Shuffle 1 min. Walk 2 min. Repeat this for 3 mi. Cool-down: Walk 5 min. **Total miles: 3** **Total kilometers: 5** **Full Marathon:** Warm-up: Walk 5 min. Shuffle 1 min. Walk 2 min. repeat this for 3 mi. Cool-down: Walk 5 min. **Total miles: 3** **Total kilometers: 5**	Walk 20–30 min. Optional for good recovery
Week 2 Building	Off	Warm-up: Walk 5 min. Shuffle 2 min. Walk 2 min. Do this 7 times Cool-down: Walk 5 min. **Total time: 38 min.**	Off	Warm-up: Walk 5 min. Shuffle 1 min. Walk 2 min. Do this 7 times Cool-down: Walk 5 min. **Total time: 31 min.**	Cross training	**Half Marathon:** Warm-up: Walk 5 min. Shuffle 1 min. Walk 2 min. Repeat this for 4 mi. Cool-down: Walk 5 min. **Total miles: 4** **Total kilometers: 6.5** **Full Marathon:** Warm-up: Walk 5 min. Shuffle 1 min. Walk 2 min. Repeat this for 4 mi. Cool-down: Walk 5 min. **Total miles: 4** **Total kilometers: 6.5**	Walk 20–30 min.
Week 3 Building	Off	Warm-up: Walk 5 min. Shuffle 3 min. Walk 2 min. Do this 7 times Cool-down: Walk 5 min. **Total time: 45 min.**	Off	Warm-up: Walk 5 min. Shuffle 2 min. Walk 2 min. Do this 6 times Cool-down: Walk 5 min. **Total time: 34 min.**	Cross training	**Half Marathon:** Warm-up: Walk 5 min. Shuffle 2 min. Walk 2 min. Repeat this for 5 mi. Cool-down: Walk 5 min. **Total miles: 5** **Total kilometers: 8** **Full Marathon:** Warm-up: Walk 5 min. Shuffle 2 min. Walk 2 min. Repeat this for 5 mi. Cool-down: Walk 5 min. **Total miles: 5** **Total kilometers: 8**	Walk 20–30 min.
Week 4 Recovery	Off	Warm-up: Walk 5 min. Shuffle 3 min. Walk 2 min. Do this 6 times Cool-down: Walk 5 min. **Total 40 min.**	Off	Warm-up: Walk 5 min. Shuffle 2 min. Walk 2 min. Do this 5 times Cool-down: Walk 5 min. **Total time: 30 min.**	Cross training	**Half Marathon:** Warm-up: Walk 5 min. Shuffle 2 min. Walk 2 min. Repeat this for 3 mi. Cool-down: Walk 5 min. **Total miles: 3** **Total kilometers: 5** **Full Marathon:** Warm-up: Walk 5 min. Shuffle 2 min. Walk 2 min. Repeat this for 4 mi. Cool-down: Walk 5 min. **Total miles: 4** **Total kilometers: 6.5**	Walk 20–30 min.

Pattern	Mon.	Tues.	Wed.	Thurs.	Fri.	Sat. Long-Run Day		Sun.
Week 5 Building: okay, no more shuffling; you're jogging now!	Off	Warm-up: Walk 5 min. Jog 3 min. Walk 1 min. Do this 9 times Cool-down: Walk 5 min. **Total time: 46 min.**	Off	Warm-up: Walk 5 min. Jog 2 min. Walk 1 min. Do this 8 times Cool-down: Walk 5 min. **Total time: 34 min.**	Cross training	**Half Marathon:** Warm-up: Walk 5 min. Jog 2 min. Walk 1 min. Repeat this for 4 mi. Cool-down: Walk 5 min. **Total miles: 4** **Total kilometers: 6.5**	**Full Marathon:** Warm-up: Walk 5 min. Jog 2 min. Walk 1 min. Repeat this for 5 mi. Cool-down: Walk 5 min. **Total miles: 5** **Total kilometers: 8**	Walk 20–30 min.
Week 6 Building	Off	Warm-up: Walk 5 min. Jog 5 min. Walk 1 min. Do this 7 times Cool-down: Walk 5 min. **Total time: 52 min.**	Off	Warm-up: Walk 5 min. Jog 3 min. Walk 1 min. Do this 7 times Cool-down: Walk 5 min. **Total time: 38 min.**	Cross training	**Half Marathon:** Warm-up: Walk 5 min. Jog 3 min. Walk 1 min. Repeat this for 5 mi. Cool-down: Walk 5 min. **Total miles: 5** **Total kilometers: 8**	**Full Marathon:** Warm-up: Walk 5 min. Jog 3 min. Walk 1 min. Repeat this for 6 mi. Cool-down: Walk 5 min. **Total miles: 6** **Total kilometers: 10**	Walk 20–30 min.
Week 7 Building	Off	Warm-up: Walk 5 min. Jog 6 min. Walk 1 min. Do this 6 times Cool-down: Walk 5 min. **Total time: 52 min.**	Off	Warm-up: Walk 5 min. Jog 4 min. Walk 1 min. Do this 6 times Cool-down: Walk 5 min. **Total time: 40 min.**	Cross training	**Half Marathon:** Warm-up: Walk 5 min. Jog 4 min. Walk 1 min. Repeat this for 6 mi. Cool-down: Walk 5 min. **Total miles: 6** **Total kilometers: 10**	**Full Marathon:** Warm-up: Walk 5 min. Jog 4 min. Walk 1 min. Repeat this for 8 mi. Cool-down: Walk 5 min. **Total miles: 8** **Total kilometers: 13**	Walk 20–30 min.
Week 8 Recovery	Off	Warm-up: Walk 5 min. Jog 4 min. Walk 1 min. Do this 6 times Cool-down: Walk 5 min. **Total time: 40 min.**	Off	Warm-up: Walk 5 min. Jog 2 min. Walk 1 min. Do this 10 times Cool-down: Walk 5 min. **Total time: 40 min.**	Cross training	**Half Marathon:** Warm-up: Walk 5 min. Jog 2 min. Walk 1 min. Repeat this for 4 mi. Cool-down: Walk 5 min. **Total miles: 4** **Total kilometers: 6.5**	**Full Marathon:** Warm-up: Walk 5 min. Jog 2 min. Walk 1 min. Repeat this for 6 mi. Cool-down: Walk 5 min. **Total miles: 6** **Total kilometers: 10**	Walk 20–30 min.

Zero to Marathon or Half Marathon in 26 Weeks

Pattern	Mon.	Tues.	Wed.	Thurs.	Fri.	Sat. Long-Run Day	Sun.
Week 9 Building	Off	Warm-up: Walk 5 min. Jog 6 min. Walk 1 min. Do this 7 times. Cool-down: Walk 5 min. **Total time: 59 min.**	Off	Warm-up: Walk 5 min. Jog 4 min. Walk 1 min. Do this 6 times. Cool-down: Walk 5 min. **Total time: 40 min.**	Cross training	**Half Marathon:** Warm-up: Walk 5 min. Jog 4 min. Walk 1 min. Repeat this for 5 mi. Cool-down: Walk 5 min. **Total miles: 5** **Total kilometers: 8** **Full Marathon:** Warm-up: Walk 5 min. Jog 4 min. Walk 1 min. Repeat this for 9 mi. Cool-down: Walk 5 min. **Total miles: 9** **Total kilometers: 14.5**	Walk 20–30 min.
Week 10 Moderate, recovery	Off	Warm-up: Walk 5 min. Jog 8 min. Walk 1 min. Do this 4 times. Cool-down: Walk 5 min. **Total time: 46 min.**	Off	Warm-up: Walk 5 min. Jog 5 min. Walk 1 min. Do this 5 times. Cool-down: Walk 5 min. **Total time: 40 min.**	Cross Training	**Half Marathon:** Warm-up: Walk 5 min. Jog 5 min. Walk 1 min. Repeat this for 4 mi. Cool-down: Walk 5 min. **Total miles: 4** **Total kilometers: 6.5** **Full Marathon:** Warm-up: Walk 5 min. Jog 5 min. Walk 1 min. Repeat this for 7 mi. Cool-down: Walk 5 min. **Total miles: 7** **Total kilometers: 11**	Walk 20–30 min.
Week 11 Building	Off	Warm-up: Walk 5 min. Jog 10 min. Walk 1 min. Do this 4 times. Cool-down: Walk 5 min. **Total time: 54 min.**	Off	Warm-up: Walk 5 min. Jog 6 min. Walk 1 min. Do this 5 times. Cool-down: Walk 5 min. **Total time: 45 min.**	Cross Training	**Half Marathon:** Warm-up: Walk 5 min. Jog 6 min. Walk 1 min. Repeat this for 6 mi. Cool-down: Walk 5 min. **Total miles: 6** **Total kilometers: 10** **Full Marathon:** Warm-up: Walk 5 min. Jog 6 min. Walk 1 min. Repeat this for 10 mi. Cool-down: Walk 5 min. **Total miles: 10** **Total kilometers: 16**	Walk 20–30 min.
Week 12 Easy, recovery	Off	Warm-up: Walk 5 min. Jog 8 min. Walk 1 min. Do this 3 times. Cool-down: Walk 5 min. **Total time: 37 min.**	Off	Warm-up: Walk 5 min. Jog 5 min. Walk 1 min. Do this 4 times. Cool-down: Walk 5 min. **Total time: 34 min.**	Cross Training	**Half Marathon:** Warm-up: Walk 5 min. Jog 5 min. Walk 1 min. Repeat this for 5 mi. Cool-down: Walk 5 min. **Total miles: 5** **Total kilometers: 8** **Full Marathon:** Warm-up: Walk 5 min. Jog 5 min. Walk 1 min. Repeat this for 8 mi. Cool-down: Walk 5 min. **Total miles: 8** **Total kilometers: 13**	Walk 20–30 min.

Pattern	Mon.	Tues.	Wed.	Thurs.	Fri.	Sat. Long-Run Day	Sun.
Week 13 Building	Off	Warm-up: Walk 5 min. Jog 10 min. Walk 1 min. Do this 4 times Cool-down: Walk 5 min. **Total time: 54 min.**	Off	Warm-up: Walk 5 min. Jog 8 min. Walk 1 min. Do this 3 times Cool-down: Walk 5 min. **Total time: 37 min.**	Cross training	**Half Marathon:** Warm-up: Walk 5 min. Jog 8 min. Walk 1 min. Repeat this for 6 mi. Cool-down: Walk 5 min. **Total miles: 6** **Total kilometers: 10** **Full Marathon:** Warm-up: Walk 5 min. Jog 8 min. Walk 1 min. Repeat this for 11 mi. Cool-down: Walk 5 min. **Total miles: 11** **Total kilometers: 18**	Walk 20–30 min.
Week 14 Moderate, recovery	Off	Warm-up: Walk 5 min. Jog 15 min. Walk 1 min. Do this 2 times Cool-down: Walk 5 min. **Total time: 42 min.**	Off	Warm-up: Walk 5 min. Jog 10 min. Walk 1 min. Do this 3 times Cool-down: Walk 5 min. **Total time: 43 min.**	Cross training	**Half Marathon:** Warm-up: Walk 5 min. Jog 10 min. Walk 1 min. Repeat this for 5 mi. Cool-down: Walk 5 min. **Total miles: 5** **Total kilometers: 8** **Full Marathon:** Warm-up: Walk 5 min. Jog 10 min. Walk 1 min. Repeat this for 9 mi. Cool-down: Walk 5 min. **Total miles: 9** **Total kilometers: 14.5**	Walk 20–30 min.
Week 15 Building	Off	Warm-up: Walk 5 min Jog 15 min. Walk 1 min. Do this 3 times Cool-down: Walk 5 min. **Total time: 58 min.**	Off	Warm-up: Walk 5 min. Jog 10 min. Walk 1 min. Do this 3 times Cool-down: Walk 5 min. **Total time: 43 min.**	Cross training	**Half Marathon:** Warm-up: Walk 5 min. Jog 10 min. Walk 1 min. Repeat this for 6 mi. or a 10-km event Cool-down: Walk 5 min. **Total miles: 6** **Total kilometers: 10** **Full Marathon:** Warm-up: Walk 5 min. Jog 10 min. Walk 1 min. Repeat this for 13 m. or a half-marathon event Cool-down: Walk 5 min. **Total miles: 13** **Total kilometers: 21**	Walk 20–30 min.
Week 16 Easy, recovery	Off	Warm-up: Walk 5 min. Jog 15 min. Walk 1 min. Do this 2 times Cool-down: Walk 5 min. **Total time: 42 min.**	Off	Warm-up: Walk 5 min. Jog 10 min. Walk 1 min. Do this 2 times Cool-down: Walk 5 min. **Total time: 32 min.**	Cross training	**Half Marathon:** Warm-up: Walk 5 min. Jog 10 min. Walk 1 min. Repeat this for 4 mi. Cool-down: Walk 5 min. **Total miles: 4** **Total kilometers: 6.5** **Full Marathon:** Warm-up: Walk 5 min. Jog 10 min. Walk 1 min. Repeat this for 8 mi. Cool-down: Walk 5 min. **Total miles: 8** **Total Kilometers: 13**	Walk 20–30 min.

Zero to Marathon or Half Marathon in 26 Weeks

Pattern	Mon.	Tues.	Wed.	Thurs.	Fri.	Sat. Long-Run Day	Sun.
Week 17 Building	Off	Warm-up: Walk 5 min. Jog 20 min. Walk 1 min. Do this 2 times Cool-down: Walk 5 min. **Total time: 52 min.**	Off	Warm-up: Walk 5 min. Jog 15 min. Walk 1 min. Do this 2 times Cool-down: Walk 5 min. **Total time: 42 min.**	Cross training	**Half Marathon:** Warm-up: Walk 5 min. Jog 15 min. Walk 1 min. Repeat this for 8 mi. Cool-down: Walk 5 min. **Total miles: 8** **Total kilometers: 13** **Full Marathon:** Warm-up: Walk 5 min. Jog 15 min. Walk 1 min. Repeat this for 14 mi. Cool-down: Walk 5 min. **Total miles: 14** **Total kilometers: 22.5**	Walk 20–30 min.
Week 18 Moderate, recovery	Off	Warm-up: Walk 5 min. Jog 20 min. Walk 1 min. Cool-down: Walk 5 min. **Total time: 31 min.**	Off	Warm-up: Walk 5 min. Jog 15 min. Walk 1 min. Do this 2 times Cool-down: Walk 5 min. **Total time: 42 min.**	Cross training	**Half Marathon:** Warm-up: Walk 5 min. Jog 15 min. Walk 1 min. Repeat this for 5 mi. Cool-down: Walk 5 min. **Total miles: 5** **Total kilometers: 8** **Full Marathon:** Warm-up: Walk 5 min. Jog 15 min. Walk 1 min. Repeat this for 10 mi. Cool-down: Walk 5 min. **Total miles: 10** **Total kilometers: 16**	Walk 20–30 min.
Week 19 Building	Off	Warm-up: Walk 5 min. Jog 20 min. Walk 1 min. Do this 2 times Cool-down: Walk 5 min. **Total time: 52 min.**	Off	Warm-up: Walk 5 min. Jog 15 min. Walk 1 min. Do this 2 times Cool-down: Walk 5 min. **Total time: 42 min.**	Cross training	**Half Marathon:** Warm-up: Walk 5 min. Jog 15 min. Walk 1 min. Repeat this for 9 mi. Cool-down: Walk 5 min. **Total miles: 9** **Total kilometers: 14.5** **Full Marathon:** Warm-up: Walk 5 min. Jog 15 min. Walk 1 min. Repeat this for 16 mi. Cool-down: Walk 5 min. **Total miles: 16** **Total kilometers: 25.5**	Walk 20–30 min.
Week 20 Easy, recovery	Off	Warm-up: Walk 5 min. Jog 30 min. Cool-down: Walk 5 min. **Total time: 40 min.**	Off	Warm-up: Walk 5 min. Jog 10 min. Walk 1 min. Do this 2 times Cool-down: Walk 5 min. **Total time: 32 min.**	Cross training	**Half Marathon:** Warm-up: Walk 5 min. Jog 10 min. Walk 1 min. Repeat this for 4 mi. Cool-down: Walk 5 min. **Total miles: 4** **Total kilometers: 6.5** **Full Marathon:** Warm-up: Walk 5 min. Jog 10 min. Walk 1 min. Repeat this for 8 mi. Cool-down: Walk 5 min. **Total miles: 8** **Total kilometers: 13**	Walk 20–30 min.

Pattern	Mon.	Tues.	Wed.	Thurs.	Fri.	Sat. Long Run Day	Sun.
Week 21 Building, working on mileage preparation	Off	Warm-up: Walk 5 min. Jog 30 min. Cool-down: Walk 5 min. **Total time: 40 min.**	Off	Warm-up: Walk 5 min. Jog 20 min. Cool-down: Walk 5 min. **Total time: 30 min.**	Cross training	**Full Marathon:** Warm-up: Walk 5 min. Jog 20 min. Walk 1 min. Repeat this for 9 mi. Cool-down: Walk 5 min. **Total miles: 9** **Total kilometers: 14.5**	Walk 20–30 min.
Week 22 Recovery	Off	Warm-up: Walk 5 min. Jog 15 min. Walk 1 min. Do this 2 times Cool-down: Walk 5 min. **Total time: 42 min.**	Off	Warm-up: Walk 5 min. Jog 30 min. Cool-down: Walk 5 min. **Total time: 40 min.**	Cross training	**Half Marathon:** Warm-up: Walk 5 min. Jog 30 min. Walk 1 min. Repeat this for 5 mi. Cool-down: Walk 5 min. (Event practice! Set up water stations at approx. distances of those of the event.) **Total miles: 5** **Total kilometers: 8**	Walk 20–30 min.
						Full Marathon: Warm-up: Walk 5 min. Jog 30 min. Walk 1 min. Repeat this for 10 mi. Cool-down: Walk 5 min. (Event practice! Set up water stations at approx. distances of those of the event.) **Total miles: 10** **Total kilometers: 16**	
Week 23 Peak mileage	Off	Warm-up: Walk 5 min. Jog 30 min. Cool-down: Walk 5 min. **Total time: 40 min.**	Off	Warm-up: Walk 5 min. Jog 20 min. Cool-down: Walk 5 min. **Total time: 30 min.**	Cross training	**Half Marathon:** Warm-up: Walk 5 min. Jog 20 min. Walk 1 min. Repeat this for 11 mi. Cool-down: Walk 5 min. **Total miles: 11** **Total kilometers: 18**	Walk 20–30 min.
						Full Marathon: Warm-up: Walk 5 min. Jog 20 min. Walk 1 min. Repeat this for 20 mi. Cool-down: Walk 5 min. **Total miles: 20** **Total kilometers: 32**	
Week 24 Moderate, recovery	Off	Warm-up: Walk 5 min. Jog 20 min. Walk 1 min. Do this 2 times Cool-down: Walk 5 min. **Total time: 52 min.**	Off	Warm-up: Walk 5 min. Jog 20 min. Cool-down: Walk 5 min. **Total time: 30 min.**	Cross training	**Half Marathon:** Warm-up: Walk 5 min. Jog 30 min. Walk 1 min. Repeat this for 8 mi. Cool-down: Walk 5 min. **Total miles: 8** **Total kilometers: 13**	Walk 20–30 min.
						Full Marathon: Warm-up: Walk 5 min. Jog 30 min. Walk 1 min. Repeat this for 16 m. Cool-down: Walk 5 min. **Total miles: 16** **Total kilometers: 25.5**	

Zero to Marathon or Half Marathon in 26 Weeks

Pattern	Mon.	Tues.	Wed.	Thurs.	Fri.	Sat. Long-Run Day	Sun.
Week 25 Easy, recovery	Off	Warm-up: Walk 5 min. Jog 30 min. Cool-down: Walk 5 min. **Total time: 40 min.**	Off	Warm-up: Walk 5 min. Jog 15 min. Cool-down: Walk 5 min. **Total time: 25 min.**	Cross training	**Half Marathon:** Warm-up: Walk 5 min. Jog 15 min. Walk 1 min. Repeat this for 4 mi. Cool-down: Walk 5 min. **Total miles: 4** **Total kilometers: 6.5** **Full Marathon:** Warm-up: Walk 5 min. Jog 15 min. Walk 1 min. Repeat this for 8 mi. Cool-down: Walk 5 min. **Total miles: 8** **Total kilometers: 13**	Walk 20–30 min.
Week 26 You did it! Easy, recovery, rest	Off	Warm-up: Walk 5 min. Jog 30 min. Cool-down: Walk 5 min. **Total time: 40 min.**	Off	Warm-up: Walk 5 min. Jog 20 min. Cool-down: Walk 5 min. **Total time: 30 min.**	Cross training	**Half Marathon:** EVENT DAY! Remember to warm up: Walk 5 min. Jog 30 min. Walk 1 min. Jog 20 min. Walk 1 min. Jog 15 min. Walk 1 min. Choose one of the above or do a combination as you feel and repeat for the HALF MARATHON! **Full Marathon:** EVENT DAY! Remember to warm up: Walk 5 min. Jog 30 min. Walk 1 min. Jog 20 min. Walk 1 min. Jog 15 min. Walk 1 min. Choose one of the above or do a combination as you feel and repeat for the FULL MARATHON!	Walk 20–30 min. Congrats!

Index

health benefits of running, 3, 7, 17, 29. *See also* cardiovascular system

health care providers, 160; when to consult, 14, 19, 94, 103, 139, 140, 170–71, 186, 192. *See also* sport medicine physicians

hill running, 29, 70–71, 196

hip flexor, 35, 122, 124, 125; stretch, 202

hitting the wall, 183–84

Hodge, Derek, 132

hydration, 7, 85, 87–88, 102, 140, 184, 188, 192. *See also* dehydration; overhydration

hyponatremia. *See* overhydration

icing of injuries, 162

iliotibial band, 161; stretch, 201

illness and running, 17–18. *See also* colds; injuries

injuries, 5, 18, 52, 67, 75, 155–76; common, 160–62, 167–68; preventing, 12–13, 28–29, 40, 121–25, 155–57, 193; resuming activity after, 159–60, 165, 171; RICE treatment, 162–63

iron, 92, 94, 103

Joy, Liz, 138, 139, 145

Kanuka, Lynn, 40

knees, 161, 162, 163, 164, 201

logbook, 32, 54–55, 64–65, 68, 82, 95, 199

Macintyre, Jim, 158, 159

Moore, Phil, 19–20, 23

motivation, 9, 30, 31–32, 35, 40, 72, 75, 78, 82, 105–19, 130, 135, 137, 170, 182–83, 199. *See also* goal setting; logbook

muscles. *See* adaptation of body to running; cooling down; core muscle strength; soreness; stiffness; stretching and strengthening; warming up

nausea, 38, 89, 169

Nordahl, Karen, 138–39

nutrition, 7, 32–33, 37–38, 85–87, 88–89, 91–103, 151, 160; pre- and post-race, 97–98, 184–86, 192; vegetarian, 86, 94, 185

orthopedic problems, 15, 16, 138

orthotics, 161, 163–64

overhydration, 89–91

overload principle, 55–56

overtraining, 10, 27, 36, 40, 49, 158, 170–71

pace, 37, 39, 41, 44, 49, 52, 53, 54, 58, 60–61, 64, 82–84, 90, 125, 134, 156, 174, 180, 183; chart, 83

Parkinson, Nicky, 153, 154

PARmed-X (Physical Activity Readiness Medical Examination), 14

PAR-Q (Physical Activity Readiness Questionnaire), 13–14, 203

Parsons, Dallas, 85, 87, 88, 91–92, 93, 95, 98, 100–101, 184

partners, running, 37, 38, 74–75, 119, 130, 135–37, 144, 156, 166, 198–99. *See also* dogs, running with

patello-femoral syndrome, 161

physicians. *See* health care providers; sport medicine physicians

plantar fasciitis, 161

pool running, 75, 128–30, 171, 173, 174, 175

Porter, Derek, 25

posture, 43, 64, 123, 124, 126, 166

pregnancy and lactation, 12, 86, 137–41, 145

Prochaska, J.O., 107

pronation, 20, 23, 61, 159, 161

psychology of running, 30, 78, 81–82, 105–19, 177, 181–83. *See also* burnout; goal setting; motivation

quadriceps stretch, 201

race day, 81–84, 177–90; jitters, 41, 75, 181–82, 189; predicting time, 82–84, 180–81, 189–90

rest and recovery, 39–40, 51, 56, 162–63, 169, 170, 192–94, 199
rhythm, 62, 64, 125, 126–27
RICE, 161, 162–63
runner's knee, 161
Runner's World magazine, 4
Running USA, 12, 39

safety, 41–42, 45, 132, 135
Savege, Jill, 26
Sedgwick, Whitney, 112, 113–14, 116, 117
shin splints, 161
shoes. *See* footwear
shoulder and chest stretch, 202
shuffle, 52, 53, 54, 58, 60–61, 64, 90
sleep, 3, 7, 45, 58, 62, 65, 74, 141, 169, 178
Smith, Trent, 15–16, 144, 147
soreness, 28, 29, 38, 40, 46, 62, 75, 122, 149, 155, 160, 170, 193
sport bras, 23, 25–26, 140–41, 168, 180
sport medicine physicians, when to consult, 7, 10, 15, 122, 149, 160, 162, 163, 165
sport medicine practitioners, types of, 160
stamina, 14, 29, 30, 51, 52, 55, 70, 123, 127, 128, 191
Steinfeld, Allan, 12
Stern, Joseph, 163
stiffness, 28, 29, 40, 124, 191, 194
stretching and strengthening, 12–13, 18, 35, 67, 121–25, 159, 161, 166; exercises, 34–35, 201–2
supination, 20, 23, 61, 159
surfaces for running, 15, 29, 44, 75, 158–59, 161, 175, 177
sweating, 24, 87, 89, 168, 169

Taunton, Jack, 31, 89, 90, 123, 160
technique, running, 42–43, 52, 64, 71, 113, 121, 123, 125–26, 166. *See also* shuffle
tendons, 16, 44, 46, 52, 67, 125, 158, 161, 163
tibial stress syndrome, 161
time. *See* race day: predicting time; when to run

Titizian, Raffi, 124
trail running, 15, 29, 75, 119, 158–59, 174, 175
training log. *See* logbook
training schedules, 10, 27, 28–29, 30–32, 35–41, 45–47, 53, 54–56, 61, 109, 135–37, 156–57. *See also* 26-week training program
26-week training program, 50–81; charts, 59, 63, 66, 69, 73, 77, 80, 204–10

urine, 103, 192

walking, 4–5, 52, 64
walk/running, 4, 5, 7, 10, 14, 17–18, 27, 31, 36, 50, 53, 111, 138–39, 145, 148
warming up, 34–35, 46, 53, 125, 160, 174, 180, 187
watches, 46, 53, 130
water. *See* hydration
water running, 75, 128–30, 171, 173, 174, 175
weather, 23–25, 88, 90, 100–101, 178, 187, 192, 193
weight. control, 3, 7, 17, 95–97, 102; overweight and running, 13, 15, 16, 28, 106, 122; weight loss from running, 88, 101, 170
when to run, 32, 45–46, 61, 142
women runners, 20, 131–33, 145; pregnancy and lactation, 12, 137–41; safety, 41–42, 45, 132, 135; sport bras, 23, 25–26, 140–41, 168, 180

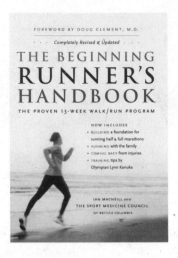